When God Stood Up

Hey Karl!
Great job.

Jim Cantelon

When God Stood Up

A Christian Response to AIDS in Africa

James Cantelon

BICENTENNIAL
1807
WILEY
2007
BICENTENNIAL

John Wiley & Sons Canada, Ltd.

National Library of Canada Cataloguing in Publication Data

Cantelon, James
    When God stood up : a Christian response to AIDS in Africa / James Cantelon.

Includes index.
ISBN: 978-0-470-83927-0

    1. AIDS (Disease)—Religious aspects—Christianity. 2. Church work with orphans—Africa. 3. Church work with widows—Africa. 4. Church work with the sick—Africa. I. Title.

BV4460.7.C36 2006   261.8'321969792   C2006-906451-2

Scripture quotations from the Old Testament, with some exceptions, are taken from the HOLY BIBLE, NEW INTERNATIONAL VERSION ®. NIV®. Copyright© 1973, 1978, 1984 by International Bible Society. Used by permission of Zondervan. All rights reserved.

Scripture quotations from the New Testament, with some exceptions, are taken from the *Holy Bible*, New Living Translation, copyright© 1996, 2004. Used by permission of Tyndale House Publishers, Inc., Carol Stream, Illinois 60188. All rights reserved

Production Credits:
Cover design: Ian Koo
Interior text design: Tegan Wallace
Printer: EPAC

John Wiley & Sons Canada, Ltd.
6045 Freemont Blvd.
Mississauga, Ontario
L5R 4J3

Printed in the United States

3 4 5 6 7 EPAC 14 13 12 11 10

To Kathy

Table of Contents

Acknowledgements

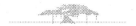

I would like to gratefully acknowledge the contributions of Dr. Testfai Yacob of Ethiopia's Kale Heywet Church, who encouraged me to write this book; Dr. Brian Stiller, who led me to Wiley Publishers; Mr. Don Loney, who fine-tuned the manuscript; and to Kathy, my wife, for her tireless efforts in assisting me throughout the project.

Abbreviations of
Biblical References

Gen.	Genesis	*Zech.*	Zechariah
Ex.	Exodus	*Mal.*	Malachi
Lev.	Leviticus	*Mt.*	Matthew
Num.	Numbers	*Mk.*	Mark
Deut.	Deuteronomy	*Lk.*	Luke
Josh.	Joshua	*Jn.*	John
Judg.	Judges	*Acts.*	Acts
Ru.	Ruth	*Rom.*	Romans
1 Sam.	1 Samuel	*1 Cor.*	1 Corinthians
2 Sam.	2 Samuel	*2 Cor.*	2 Corinthians
1 Ch.	1 Chronicles	*Eph.*	Ephesians
2 Ch.	2 Chronicles	*1 Thess.*	1 Thessalonians
Ps.	Psalms	*2 Thess.*	2 Thessalonians
Prov.	Proverbs	*Heb.*	Hebrews
Isa.	Isaiah	*Jas.*	James
Jer.	Jeremiah	*1 Pet.*	1 Peter
Lam.	Lamentations	*2 Pet.*	2 Peter
Ezek.	Ezekiel	*1 Jn.*	1 John
Dan.	Daniel	*Rev.*	Revelation
Hos.	Hosea		
Am.	Amos		
Mic.	Micah		

Introduction

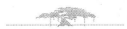

I've always admired the biblical Job. There he was, totally devastated by the loss of his entire family, fortune, and health; sitting on a dunghill; scraping his boils; surrounded by his best friends, all doing their best to accuse him of sin. And, as these "comforters" droned on, trying to accommodate Job's sufferings to their world view, Job looked past these space-time philosophies to the world beyond and said: "I know that my redeemer lives." He was so convinced of this savior God that he even stated: "Though He slay me, yet will I trust in Him."

Contrast this otherworldly detachment to that of his earth-bound wife: "Curse God and die!" Job didn't rebuke her. For all we know he took her hand, fully empathetic to her sorrow at their mutual loss, and silently comforted her. He saw what she couldn't see and had compassion. What a man! I've always wanted to be like him.

Imagine my disappointment, then, when I discovered in Africa that I'm not at all like him. Indeed, I'm not even close. I don't even have the stature of a "comforter." Bluntly and brutally put, I'm a "Job's wife."

This discovery, which has been underscored several times since, first occurred in January 2002, in a shantytown in South Africa. I was standing with a widow outside her home. "Home," by the way, needs qualification—it was a rusty tin-sheeting enclosure, with dirt for a floor, and an unstable sheet of corrugated fiberglass for a roof. It housed eighteen orphans and this bone-thin, weary, overextended woman. She was weeping.

Another orphan had been brought to her that morning. Like the others, this little one belonged to the widow's extended family; this time, a niece had died of HIV/AIDS, and the widow's home was the only option for the young child. She wept from the sorrow and the stress of it all. Compounding her anguish was the fact that the only wage-earner in her home was the fourteen-year-old boy who made twenty-five cents a day herding cattle. He had just died, too. HIV/AIDS is no respecter of people or of need.

"I just can't take it anymore," she cried, "I have nothing, no one, no hope. I just want to die." Then she paused, as if listening to an inner conversation. She glanced at me through her tears, and then looked heavenward. Lifting her emaciated hands to the sky, she said, in a whisper, "Ah, but I do have hope. I put my trust in my heavenly Father." I was in the presence of a modern-day Job.

The impact on me was crushing. It wasn't the hopelessness, the despair, the abject poverty. It was the faith. Her faith, not mine. Especially not mine. Because my immediate reaction, inwardly, was, "What have you got to bless God about? Curse God and die!"

I'm not proud of this. But at that moment I realized with naked clarity that my faith was filtered by Western comfort and entitlement. I was just a visitor on her planet. I'd never seen such faith anywhere in North America or Europe. I was standing next to a saint and I felt unworthy. So utterly unworthy.

Then I felt angry. Angry at myself, at my consumer faith, at poverty, at injustice, at HIV/AIDS. A flood of passionate impulses suddenly awakened within me, all fighting for control. I wanted to lash out, weep, curse, preach, explode, repent, grovel, escape. But a cool certainty rose above my internal conflict—my earlier "calling" to fight HIV/AIDS had been real. I was going to light a candle rather than curse the darkness. The greatest challenge of my life lay ahead. I would join the army of those fighting for the greatest victims of HIV/AIDS—the orphan and the widow.

In Chapter 3 I'll tell the story of how this "calling" came to be. I was aware from the outset that there was more to a vocation than a mere call to action. There had to be both vision and mission, strategy and action, passion and faithfulness. In other words, youthful energy had to be tempered with mature experience. There had to be initiative, follow through, accountability, and measurability. Maybe this is why the biggest chapter of my life opened at age fifty-two. The wine had to mature before being poured out.

What you're about to read is not the work of a "do-gooder." The scope of the horrors of the HIV/AIDS pandemic is too great for do-gooders. It eviscerates the merely idealistic. To even hope to make a difference in fighting humankind's greatest threat in history, one must have a sense of mandate—marching orders from above. Only strength from on high can sustain an overwhelmed and overmatched soldier. My constant companion in this battle is humility. I've never felt so inadequate or dependent. Or so little.

The HIV/AIDS pandemic is beyond fearful. Language cannot convey the devastation, so I will let stories of the valiant, the suffering, and the dying speak.

In the book I'll try to describe how the Almighty sees orphans and widows. I'll explore two of the critical ingredients in understanding the DNA of authentic faith. I also have strong words for the Church and for you, the reader, and your community.

I hope this book changes your life. My life and my wife Kathy's have been changed. And isn't that what scripture does? It's a mighty transformer wrestling with our self-absorption. So, wrestle with me. As we're changed, maybe we can change the world.

Journal

"Here I am, Lord, send me."

*W*hen I was a young boy, Africa didn't exist. Nor did Canada, America, nor the oceans for that matter. I lived in a cozy, mysterious, and exciting place called Kelvington, Saskatchewan. I didn't know it was a small town. For me it was the world.

I loved exploring that world. Just beyond the alleyway bounding our backyard was a lumber storage ground with intriguing stacks of lengths of wood arranged in rectangular piles. I spent hours climbing in, through, and over those stacks, sometimes launching myself through the air from pile to pile, sometimes landing on my stomach and getting winded as a consequence.

A little farther afield was Dempster's Pond, a slough of stagnant water that grew scummy and smelly in the heat of summer. It was a perfect destination when you were seven, especially if you had a dog. I did, and his name was Rocky. He loved water—any kind of water, anywhere, anytime. (In fact, he once jumped out of the window of our moving car when he spotted a slough, one very hot summer's day!) There were water lilies, skating spiders, bugs, tadpoles, garter snakes, snails, toads, frogs, and all of the other treasures valued by young boys. I'd make rafts out of stray pieces of wood, and pretend I was a pirate, with Rocky as first mate. We'd play all day, returning home in the late afternoon, filthy, but glowing with health. Often the first thing Mother would do was douse us both in buckets of fresh water. She said we smelled.

About a mile and a half from Dempster's, on the opposite side of town, was the town dump (or "nuisance grounds" as the locals called it).

It too was a smelly place where competing odors reached out to befoul or scorch your nostrils. Rotting food, mildewed clothing, broken glass, burning trash, dead pets(!) in various stages of wormy decay, rats, and centipedes made this place a must-visit destination for a kid. I would root about, uncovering valuables, and, even though I was young, gaining insights into the lives of the townspeople from what they had thrown away. I remember being impressed at the volume of stuff people discarded; in my home (the home of the town preacher) it seemed we threw nothing away. Making ends meet meant stretching the usefulness of seemingly every scrap.

Perhaps my favorite place to explore was the three grain elevators situated at the train station on the edge of town. The massive steam locomotives used to chug right up to these leviathans and car after car of golden grain poured down the chutes from above, as lines of wagons and trucks full of grain waited their turn to empty their cargo into the bins. What magic! The puffing and steaming of the locomotives, the colorful train engineers, the squealing of brakes laboring under the weight of tons of steel and grain, the wooden elevators—"prairie skyscrapers"—with their distinct odors of wheat and birds, the farmers with their wagons, the kids, the dogs, the transients "ridin' the rails," the bakery next to the station, the smell of freshly baked bread, coffee ... I loved it.

What I loved most was the "forbidden fruit" of climbing up inside the elevators, where a whole universe of adventure awaited. Essentially an elevator was a granary on steroids. About 60 by 60 feet square, they extended anywhere from 80 to 100 feet upwards, capped with sloping "shoulders" and a small peaked "head." Sometimes on a rainy day that head was lost in the clouds. Constructed of wood, they had a sweet-smelling presence that cracked and groaned with the wind. They sounded and felt alive.

Inside were vertical swimming-pool-sized storage bins that were accessed by baffled portals on the outside (for the grain chutes and augers) and by ladders on the inside (for men to open and close internal chutes for mixing the grain, clear stuck portals, and deal with birds' nests and rodents). The ladders were attached to the walls and climbing them was an effort physically and psychologically. Occasionally a worker would slip, or have a sudden case of vertigo, and fall into one of the bins. This would sometimes precipitate a "grain slide" and the worker would be smothered. This was why "unofficial" visits to the interior were frowned upon. The elevator manager and his employees were the only ones allowed in. Everyone else, especially seven-year-old boys, were strictly forbidden entry.

There was, however, a weak link in this impermeable fence; his name was Gus Johnson. He was a shoveler, standing in the wagons shoveling grain into buckets attached to ropes and pulleys that carried the harvest up to various levels of the elevator. He was thin, sinewy, and could work nonstop for hours at a time. It didn't seem to bother him when his sweaty body became caked with detritus, or his eyes encrusted with grain dust. I'm sure his lungs were coated too; indeed, the interior of an elevator was always dusty. Light streaming through cracks and knotholes could be seen clearly like laser-beams illuminating the polluted air. Gus was simple, toothless, and kind. And he had a soft spot for adventurers. Every time I wanted to explore, he managed to create a diversion while I crawled in through the "secret passageway" created by a few broken boards at the back. As soon as I was in, I felt the hush of another world.

I say "hush" because sometimes the diesel engine powering the rope and pulley system would be silent, the workers quietly eating in their lunchroom, the train and trucks still, and all you could hear was the twittering of the swallows and the groaning aches and pains of a large wooden building suffering the internal pressure of tons of grain testing its structural integrity. The dusty air made no sound, but in the streams of light filtering through from outside, you could see it pulsating, as if the elevator were breathing. Not far from my secret passageway the first ladder ascended. Standing at its foot I could look up, up, up through the shimmering air, all the way to the headhouse or cupola at the top. Often, as I looked up in the stillness, I would have a sense of the holy. It was as though I had entered a cathedral.

Interestingly, at other times, in the bowels of this behemoth, with ropes whizzing, pulleys screeching, tons of grain being dumped, chutes *singing, dust exploding, I still felt the spiritual quality it possessed. The headhouse was always my goal. Up there, even when the elevator was in full operation, I felt removed from the life below. I had a favorite spot, a massive beam of timber, where I could sit and think. The wonder of the machinery was eclipsed by wonder itself. As I looked out through a knothole to the whitened harvest fields stretching to the horizon, I wondered what was beyond. And what was beyond the beyond. My childish soul was beginning to stretch. Sometimes I felt like I was on the threshold of heaven.*

One early September morning I had a lot to think and wonder about. A missionary from Africa had spoken at our church the day previous, and had stayed with us that night. He had shown us a movie at service that he had taken and I had watched in total fascination. It had seemed as if I were looking at life on another planet—mud huts, dark-skinned people, strange costumes, wild dancing, exuberant church services, weird-looking food, and strange language. I had been entranced by this. When we got home from the service the missionary set up his projector and showed the movie again, this time to Mom, Dad, my brother, and me. I found it just as intoxicating the second time. And it scared me. This was a world I didn't know existed, and I felt inextricably drawn to it. It was more than Africa, it was the draw of the far horizon. That movie marked the birth of a world view, one that has continued to grow to this day.

I sat on my perch in the headhouse, pondering. Who were these people in the movie? How could they live that way? How could they be so hungry and yet so happy? And those sick kids, don't they have doctors? That kid with malaria, sweating and trembling, the missionary enters the hut, prays for him, and the next day he's well—what is healing? Does this mean they don't need doctors because God is their doctor? What about that food? Yucky-looking stuff. Gross. Does God love them like he loves us? What do they smell like? This country, Africa, must be far, far away. Must be exciting riding in that ship. What does seasick feel like? I think I'd like to go there some day. When I grow up maybe I will.

My headhouse reverie was cut short by the clanging of a bell far below. I jumped to my feet, thinking it was a fire alarm. Trapped in the immediate conflict of wanting to escape but also not wanting to be caught I began to quickly, but cautiously, descend. As I got to the third storey I heard loud voices and a desperate cry from the second-storey bin. I looked down between my feet and caught sight of two men throwing a rope.

"Hang on to this Emmit, quick! Emmit! Emmit! Here! Grab this!"

Emmit, one of the workers, had gone up to the second-storey bin for some reason, and had slipped and fallen into the grain. Like quicksand, it had engulfed him. Now, only his head and one arm were visible. He was in big trouble.

Hooking an arm through one of the rungs, I watched in horror as Emmit was suddenly covered with a slide of unstable grain. One of the men, a rope tied around his waist, jumped in after him, while the other held both ropes and called loudly for help. I could hear, and then saw, two more men scrabbling up the ladder. In a moment three of them were shouting instructions and hauling on the ropes. An eternal minute later, a bedraggled and coughing Emmit emerged, his rescuers clapping him on the back and congratulating one another on their success. They all descended to the ground floor while I remained, unseen and rooted to the spot.

After gathering myself, I silently descended to my secret passageway and crawled out into the sunshine. I was shaken. I sat for an hour or so, my back against the wall of the elevator, my head beneath the level of the long grass around me. I had seen a man almost die. And, in a heart-pounding sequence, I'd seen him rescued by his friends. My mind went back to the hymn we had sung after the missionary's film, "Rescue the Perishing." He'd said the Africans were "perishing" and we needed to "save" them. God needed laborers for the harvest field of lost people. "Would you go?" the missionary had asked.

I was only a prairie preacher's boy, seven years of age. I had only heard the "call" to Africa yesterday. I'd just seen a perishing man rescued today. Suddenly I wanted to be a rescuer. Looking up past the headhouse, way, way above me, I breathed a prayer to heaven *that I imagined was spiraling up in the thermals like the swallows wheeling overhead. I remembered my dad's sermon the week previous, and prayed, "Here I am, Lord, send me."*

Chapter 1

Righteousness and Justice:
The Foundation of Authentic Faith

*I*t's a long flight from New York to Johannesburg. For seventeen hours you hunker down in your assigned space, armrests digging into your hips, knees bumped intermittently by the person in front of you who has to get the angle of his seatback just right, flight attendants, passengers, and serving carts colliding with your over-broad shoulders jutting out into the aisle, the child behind you coughing constantly with the occasional bits of phlegmy detritus hitting your head, and ... well, you get the picture. It's a very long flight.

Kathy and I have often thought that perhaps it's good that the flight is long. Long means distance. And distance—the more of it the better—seems to justify the jolt when the very next day you find yourself in a totally foreign culture, surrounded by poverty, disease, and death. Somehow the distance, the dislocation, even the jetlag, provide the buffer you need so that the culture shock doesn't paralyze you. If it weren't for the distance, you'd feel you'd been transported to another world, a parallel universe, blind-sided by a bad dream. Those seventeen hours give you time to take some deep breaths before plunging into the deep, dark waters of Africa.

As we took the plunge for the first time (how it came to be I'll describe in a later chapter), we had no idea what lay in store. We had been to Africa before, but for a different purpose. Then it had been to speak at conferences, to inspire preachers and pastors, to share what we had learned about church ministry. Now, instead of dealing from a position of strength as veterans, my wife and I were total rookies, knowing nothing of substance about HIV/AIDS or of its victims, pursuing a vision we had for the churches of Africa, becoming Mother Teresas in the cold, black night that the pandemic had unleashed upon the continent. We had never seen an HIV-positive African. We had never held a diseased baby in our arms. We had never entered a *rondavaal*, or bathed the fevered head of someone dying a horrible death. We were just plain folk—middle-income North Americans, shaped by our culture, living with an unconscious sense of entitlement, relatively free from the sorrows that plague two-thirds of our world. We had come to do good, but had no idea what that good would be. We were in way over our heads.

Just hours after touchdown at the ultra-modern Johannesburg International Airport, we were in a rental car driving to White River in northeastern South Africa. It had been years since I'd driven on the left side of the road while on holiday in the UK, and I'd learned a valuable mantra then, one I muttered continually to myself as we drove, "Stay left, look right—stay left, look right—stay left, look right." The problem all of us North Americans have, both driving and walking, in countries with left-side driving is that we automatically look left when we stop at an intersection. Seeing all clear, we confidently step or drive out only to get clobbered by a car approaching us from the right. This is why you often see "Look Right" written into the pavement at intersections in the UK. They don't want to see their visitors t-boned.

So, staying left and looking right, Kathy and I drove a beautiful highway bounded by sweeping fields of corn, grain, and sugar cane; and, as we got closer to White River, the majestic Drakensburg mountains. In contrast to what we would see in later travels to other African countries, the vehicles on the highway were generally late models and well maintained. There were occasional "beaters" on the road belching black smoke; and, if they happened to be trucks, severely overloaded with cargo, poorly secured and out-of-plumb. Many times I held my breath passing trucks whose trailer loads were in imminent danger of falling onto the road. But overall the trip was uneventful. We stopped a couple of times at roadside service centers and were amazed at how clean and modern they were—pristine even, compared to some of their counterparts in North America. We relaxed and enjoyed the ride, unaware of the world we would enter just a few hours down the road.

Masoyi Home-Based Care

Our destination was a rural area outside of White River called Masoyi. A former "homeland" (from the apartheid era), it's a large settlement of humble homes situated on the rolling and sometimes dramatic hill country between White River and the Mozambique border. It also butts onto the southern edge of Kruger National Park, one of the most impressive game reserves in the world. About 250,000 people live in Masoyi, and, we were to learn later, 90 percent of the children there don't know who their fathers are. HIV/AIDS is running rampant in the area, and almost every one of those little hovels houses a victim of the pandemic.

Lions Head, a massive hill that looks like a male lion gazing out to the horizon, dominates Masoyi. Right at the foot of this imposing sight is a small ministry training center and state-of-the-art HIV/AIDS clinic. It was here that our hosts awaited us. The gentle volunteers of Masoyi Home-Based Care were about to introduce us to their world.

"Pasta Jim! Welcome!" exclaimed Ma Glo (Mother Gloria), the leader of the volunteers. "We're so pleased to meet you! This is your wife?"

"Yes," I answered. "This is Kathy."

"Kati!" Giving her a huge hug she took Kathy by the arm and led us into the small building where the volunteers were preparing for that day's home visits. Ma Glo introduced us to the seven women and two men. The women shyly curtsied and the men bowed as we shook hands. The African way of shaking hands is a three-part ritual: firm clasp and shake, unclasp and join hands in what I refer to as a modified arm-wrestle and shake, unclasp and clasp again in the conventional way and shake. Sometimes I forget about the three steps, withdrawing my hand after the first clasp and shake, leaving my African friends with their hands poised for clasp two. When my hand is not forthcoming, their faces betray a touch of surprise and disappointment, but they quickly recover, observing to themselves, no doubt, that we Westerners have a different handshaking protocol. Generally, though, I remember, and the three-part shake does its work; you feel like you've physically connected and the welcome is always warm.

The founder of Masoyi Home-Based Care and I had met about ten months previously in Johannesburg. He and I had started our charities at about the same time. In that first meeting we marveled at the similarity in the core values of our vision, especially the commitment to engaging local churches in the battle against HIV/AIDS and the care of its victims. We found ourselves to be kindred spirits and expected that one day we would work together. So, here we were, at his base in Masoyi, about to begin a path that would lead eventually to a strategic partnership.

Ma Glo gave us a brief orientation. She showed us the supplies stockpiled in the building. There were several piles of bagged corn-meal, about a dozen baskets of root vegetables, cans of cooking oil, and about ten shelves of rudimentary pharmaceuticals, bandages, and rubber gloves.

"This is about five days' supply," she said. "The local churches with whom we work and a few international donors make sure we're at least five days ahead of the need. Sometimes, however, we run short..." and her voice trailed off. Recovering quickly she went on.

"The cornmeal and the oil are for the homes we visit, the root vegetables are for the volunteers."

"Do you pay them anything?" Kathy asked.

"No, we don't. We can't. But we do give them enough food to keep their strength up. Home-based care is strenuous work, and most of these women are widows themselves with very small incomes. They're helping the helpless. The least we can do is help them eat."

Taking us into a small room next to the main entry, she showed us their administration setup.

"That computer is old, but it works," she said brightly. "We keep up-dated records of every home visit we make, and the condition of the people we care for. We also have a fax machine, as you can see, and that helps us connect with our overseas donors. We hope to have e-mail soon. That will be a real blessing."

Turning to a list on the wall she showed us the names and phone numbers of the local social services, hospitals, and related NGOs. "We keep in touch with all of these," she said. "We don't want to work in isolation. Plus, there are times when the social services must be informed of what we encounter, and many times we have to transport people to the hospital in Nelspruit."

"Are they cooperative?" I asked.

"Who? The hospitals?"

"Yeah. And the others. Do they respond quickly to your calls?"

"Usually. But they're understaffed, underfunded, and frankly envy our ability to recruit volunteers. Nothing like followers of Jesus responding to the broken, you know," her face beamed. "We feel the responsibility is ours to help everyone. It's just that we're a bit stretched at times."

"So, how is the day to unfold?" I asked, perhaps a bit presumptuously.

"Well, normally we're out by ten in the morning. But, we waited for you today so we'll leave at about eleven. While we waited we divided the group into pairs and have assigned each pair four homes in different parts of Masoyi. Their bags are packed with the medical supplies they'll need, and they're ready to go after we pray."

"What about the sacks of cornmeal?" Kathy asked.

"Oh, those go out in a truck once a week. They're too heavy to carry ourselves. In fact, the medical bags are heavy enough. We walk, you know."

"How far?"

"About six miles each time, but it's no problem. Everyone walks in Masoyi."

After a time of glorious singing and powerful praying (welcome to Africa!), the entire group with their heavy bags crowded with us into a van and two small pickup trucks called *bakkies*. We drove about 6 miles into the central part of Masoyi where we met up with ten more volunteers who had assembled and prepared for the day at another Masoyi Home-Based Care base. More singing. More praying. And we're off—Kathy walking with one pair of Home-Based caregivers, I with another.

Into the Fire

It's high noon, hot and dusty. We've hardly walked a mile and I'm already plodding. My head hurts. Jetlag is doing its foul work. When you're jetlagged, you feel like you did as a teenager after you'd stayed up all night on New Year's Eve. During the all-nighter you thrived on adrenaline. On way home about sunrise, you felt a dullness coming on. About ten or eleven that morning, your head felt like it weighed 30 pounds, your chest and shoulders ached, and your feet felt glued to the ground. You crashed. Went to bed and slept for ten hours, wide-awake at midnight, about to go through another cycle of dislocation. Even your eyes hurt.

Well, combine all of the above with heat, dirt, and total foreignness. I'm walking roads that most White people, let alone Westerners, have never seen. They're narrow, rough-hewn, more like riverbeds than roads, leading like alleyways through a disordered jumble of makeshift homes. Little children in oversized hand-me-down clothing watch me from the darkened doorways, caught between fascination and flight. They've been told about the White bogeymen who come to steal children away at night. I see five- and six-year-old girls with babies on their backs, and loads of water or wood on their heads, their eyes curious, their faces blank. Thin, gaunt women, bent at the waist sweeping the sandy ground in front of their houses with a short-handled broom, freeze, eyeing me with a sort of benign suspicion. One or two straighten up and wave. We wave back. African dogs are everywhere. In the West we're used to various breeds. Here only one breed prevails—it looks like a cross between a wild dog and a rat. Short, tan-colored fur, large ears, pointy face, pointy tail, thin, really thin, always hungry, never playing, avoiding people like they're avoiding a kick, never friendly, looking like canine wraiths.

"What do they eat?" I ask my companions.

"Rats, snakes, garbage, whatever they can steal."

"Do you like dogs?"

"No."

"Do they have names?"

"No. Maybe. Sometimes."

"So why do you have them?"

"Because they're there. Like trees or weeds. Plus they keep the rats out of our homes."

My companions are Marcus and Naomi. Marcus is a student at the college, and has qualifications as a nurse's aide. Naomi wants to be a nurse. She just doesn't have the money for university. They're both young and sweet and care a lot about the victims of HIV/AIDS. They may not be able to give expert care, but they're very able and willing to give their hearts. In them I see hope for the future of home-based care. There will always be widows willing to volunteer, but these two will be able one day, in the prime of their lives, to train and supervise volunteers. We've just got to get Naomi and others like her the training she needs now. A few dollars invested in her university education will bear huge dividends in the future.

Our first stop. We walk down a steep hill to a cement-block structure with rusty tin secured to the flat roof with large stones, one or two cement blocks, and an old car tire. An elderly woman is bent over an open fire, stirring something in a charcoal-black pot. She looks up, acknowledging us with a faint nod of her head, and motions us over to the door. This cool welcome, if welcome at all, is something I see over and over again as the years pass. I still can't figure it out. Why would you not receive someone warmly who has come to help you care for your dying loved one? My only thought is that it's because they're so worn out. Caring for someone who is dying is a relentless task. There's no relief. There's no hope. There's no thanks. So maybe the granny has no energy left. Not even enough to crack a smile. Maybe she's more dead than alive.

The patient is her twenty-seven-year-old son. He lies in the kitchen of the two-room house, his bed the back seat taken from an abandoned car. His head and his feet extend over the ends of the car seat. His face is gaunt, cheekbones and eyes protruding, ribs prominent, legs as thin as sticks. He wears only the bottoms of undersized, striped pajamas. His lips are cracked, and his skin is covered with sores. He lifts his head momentarily as we enter, then with a sigh lowers it again. His name is Nathan, and he looks like a very old, sick man.

Naomi sees the cracked lips and immediately goes outside to get water. Marcus begins to apply topical cream to his sores. As he does so, he talks with Nathan in a quiet, affirming manner. Nathan responds weakly, but at least he responds. Marcus questions him about his aches, pains, and fever, making notes in the log as Nathan painfully answers. The granny stays outside. I hear Naomi calmly but strongly urging her to keep Nathan hydrated. Marcus introduces me to Nathan. I take his hand—probably the hottest hand I've ever touched.

"He's burning up!" I remark to Marcus.

"Yeah, I know. He needs some *panado* (South African aspirin)." "Here, Nathan, take this." Nathan lifts his head with effort and swallows the pills with a cup of water that Naomi has just brought in. He swallows with excruciating difficulty, choking and coughing, bloody phlegm emerging form the corners of his mouth. While Marcus deals with this, Naomi calls the granny in, and kindly lectures her about Nathan's need for water, *panado*, and topical relief of his sores. She gives her the pills and the cream, and sternly says, "We'll be back next week. I hope I don't find him thirsty again." (Maybe this is why she gave us no welcome, I think.) They ask me to pray. I pray for comfort, for relief, for faith. The words come from my mouth. My heart is empty. I feel like a phony. I'm overcome with sorrow. What if this boy was one of my own two sons?

Over the next few hours I see sorrow on sorrow. Gladys, seventeen years old, hollow-cheeked and thin, sits in the doorway of her one-room cement shack, a plastic bag of breadcrumbs at her side, her only food for the day, too weak to do anything but shuffle over to the thorn tree to relieve herself. Dorcas, twenty, lies on her plastic-covered mattress, ugly bed sores on her bony hips, her one-year-old son crying for food. Emmanuel, all by himself, a thirty-year-old skeleton, walks slowly to the toilet, stopping to throw up on the way. We return to base. I'm destroyed.

Kathy returns a few minutes later. She's distraught. We silently move to the shade of a two-barreled water tower and she says, "Jim, there's this young mother, three kids, lying on her bed, unable to get up. I'm sure she'll die tonight. Her kids are so little, so helpless, sitting there with her, crying. Ma Glo has got to get her to the clinic. Now!"

With that, she half-runs over to Ma Glo, who has just returned from her rounds. I see Kathy urgently speaking to her, her face lined with concern, her hands gesticulating, her body taut with focus and determination. Ma Glo takes out her cellphone. I see her talking for a minute or two. She turns to Kathy, says something, and Kathy returns to me.

"They're sending a truck. Ma Glo is going to get her to the clinic. I hope it's not too late."

We drive back to base number one. Ma Glo rides with us. We talk about the day. She tells us this is just another of an endless day of sorrows. "We do what we can," she sighs, "for Jesus's sake." We drop her and the others off and drive to our country guesthouse. We eat in silence, the food wooden and tasteless. *What have we gotten ourselves into?*

The Televangelist and the Teddy Bear

A fourteen-year-old girl in Lusaka, Zambia is talking to a journalist about HIV/AIDS.

"My girlfriends and I have discovered how to avoid HIV/AIDS," she says.

"Really?" says the journalist. "How?"

"Don't sleep with the pastor," she replies.

What! Don't sleep with the pastor? The man who "shepherds" the flock? The man of God? The man who above all men should be trusted, with whom all little girls should feel safe? Don't sleep with the pastor? Where's the righteousness?

And where's the justice? The pastor as predator? The pastor as transmitter of death? The pastor as abuser? When and how did the confession "I am a Christian" lose its meaning? And where is the heavenly father and judge in all of this? Has he somehow vanished from the landscape?

I first heard this story when we started our work with HIV/AIDS in January 2000. It troubled me deeply then; it troubles me now. And it evokes a memory of similar disquiet back in the 1980s when the Israeli press asked me to give them a press conference on the American televangelist scandals.

"Mr. Swaggart" and "Mr. Bakker" were mentioned by name only once—and with respect. The Israelis seemed more tuned to human frailty and compassion in their coverage of the scandals than were the North American press. What intrigued them was Americans' shock at the behavior of these televangelists. When I observed that we expect preachers specifically and all Christians generally to practise what they preach, one of the reporters said, "Yes, but men, be they preachers or no, need sex, right?" When I responded, "Your own scriptures teach that sex is exclusively for marriage," they laughed. Politely. But they laughed. As far as they were concerned, the big story wasn't about sexual peccadilloes, but about the unreal moral code of Christians—a code that was flaunted in the pulpit, and denied in the bedroom, by preachers who showed their true colors in the dark. I think what troubled me the most about this exchange was the Israeli press's view that a high view of sex was aberrant, and that the televangelists had done us all a favor by stripping off the veneer of moral rectitude and exposing good old-fashioned hypocrisy.

One of the reporters scored a huge point when he said, "Aren't these televangelists the guys who manipulate our scriptures and come up with prophecies about Israel and the end of the world? You know, sometimes they make us think. Now, I don't know what to think."

This hit home for I'd just been dealing with "end-time" weirdness that week. A woman from Texas had dropped by my office. She had that wild look in her eye that I had seen countless times before in Jerusalem. And like so many others before her, she had had a "revelation" that God wanted her to go to the Holy City. But her "calling" had been a bit more novel than most.

"You know, Pastor, I was walking home from my church in Houston a few Sundays ago, and, just as I approached my house, I saw my daughter's teddy bear on the sidewalk, so I bent down to pick it up, and you know what, Pastor? The teddy bear spoke to me!" I was speechless.

"And you probably want to know what it said?" she asked. I nodded dumbly.

"'Get thee to Jerusalem and become a watchman on the walls,'" it said.

"So here I am," she exclaimed triumphantly. "What should I do now?"

I won't tell you what I thought, or said (although I did wonder irreverently if the teddy bear had spoken with a Texan accent). But it was one of those "watchman-on-the-walls," wide-eyed, out-of-focus, glazed, true-believer conversations that I never invited but often fell into because of my position as pastor of the largest Protestant evangelical church in Israel. Jerusalem as a mecca attracts "flakes" like food attracts flies, and I've had more than my share land on me. People call this weirdness "The Jerusalem Syndrome." Call it what you will, religious zealotry knows no bounds. It seems there are no theological checks and balances to rein it in.

So the Texas teddy bear and the televangelist fiasco pushed me over the edge. I called in my staff after that and declared that I didn't care how long it would take, or how hard I would have to work, I was going to study every prophetic passage in the Old Testament. I wanted to see if there was a crystalized message, a common theme or denominator, a recurring thread that would bring some sanity, some consistency, some integrity to the interpretation of biblical writings about the "end of days." I'd had it with boneheads.

Distilling the Message

It took a year, but I discovered that there is a common message in Old Testament prophetic passages. (Before I tell you what it is, you should know that prophecy in the Bible is more about "forth-telling" than "fore-telling." There are occasional future themes in Old Testament prophecy, but generally a prophecy is given by a "prophet" concerned with a present-day issue. He or she speaks, usually to the national leadership, about a value, circumstance, cultural trend, or political/religious tendency that has gone missing or is in need of correction. The "word" is often like a fist to the jaw, but always ends on a positive note.) That message is a call to Israel to return to the right relationship with God and the right relationship with neighbor. Or, to put it succinctly, the Old Testament prophets want us to be righteous and just.

The prophetic passages of the Old Testament are many and varied. There are the "major" prophetic books like Isaiah, Jeremiah, and Ezekiel; the "minor" works like Amos, Hosea, and Habakkuk (to name a few), and then there are sporadic prophetic words—sometimes a paragraph or two, sometimes a sentence—that occur in "non-prophetic" books like Genesis or Deuteronomy, and even in the Psalms. The core concerns of most prophetic messages generally refer to one of four "sins": idolatry (a low view of God), adultery (a low view of neighbor), neglect of the poor (again, a low view of neighbor), and the shedding of innocent blood (once more, a low view of neighbor). The sin of idolatry is usually seen as a process. Israel "forgets" the name of the Lord and then replaces him with someone or something else. They settle for a dumb idol, and in so doing are guilty of a low view of God (the sin of unrighteousness). The sins of adultery, neglect of the poor, and shedding innocent blood put self before other, and betray a low view of neighbor (the sin of injustice). The call of scripture is that Israel return to a "high view of God" (righteousness) and a "high view of neighbor" (justice). The focus of righteousness is love for God. The focus of justice is love for neighbor. And if someone in Old Testament times were to ask the question, "Who is my neighbor?", the answer would be, "start with the alien, the orphan, and the widow."

Jesus himself captured the prophetic call of the Old Testament when he responded to a young lawyer seeking to know what it was that God expected of him. "What's the bottom line of God's expectation?" was the essential question. Jesus's answer? It's recorded three times in the gospels, and here it is in summary: "Israel has one God, and he is one. Love him with everything you are and have. Love your neighbor the same way—and, yes, love yourself that way too." And, to emphasize the point, he goes on to say, "There is no law of God greater than righteousness [love for God] and justice [love for neighbor]. All of God's expectations of you are there. Be righteous and just and you will live both now and in the everlasting world that awaits" (see Mk. 12:28–31; Mt. 22:34–40; Lk. 10:25–28). Notice there's no call to religiosity or dogma here. It is purely a call to love of God and neighbor. Static compliance to the letter of the law gives way to a fluid pursuit of the spirit of the law where righteousness and justice are the fuel of freedom.

Here is just a taste of those Old Testament prophetic words: "Righteousness and justice are the foundation of your throne; love and faithfulness go before you" (Ps. 89:14). "I will make justice the measuring line and righteousness the plumb line..." (Isa. 28:17). Everything that God builds (in this case, "Zion," v. 16), he builds on the foundation and through the lens of righteousness and justice. None of us would ever enter a building or cross a bridge if we didn't believe that the builders knew and practised proper measurement and plumb. Without these skills the building collapses and people inside die; the bridge gives way and cars plunge into the canyon. So too righteousness and justice are critical to sustainability.

By the way, Isaiah also presents the obverse: when referring to God's coming judgment of the nation of Edom, Isaiah says, "God will stretch out over Edom the measuring line of chaos and the plumb line of desolation" (34:11b). So we choose: will it be righteousness or desolation, justice or chaos? Two of the "classic" prophetic words come from the "minor" prophets Amos and Micah: "Let justice roll on like a river, righteousness like a never-failing stream" (Am. 5:24)! "He has showed you, O man, what is good. And what does the Lord require of you? To act justly and to love mercy and to walk humbly with your God" (Mic. 6:8). In the materialism of Amos's and Micah's day, Israel had forgotten their God, were arrogant, and abusive of their neighbors, who "trample the needy ... buying the poor with silver and the needy for a pair of sandals" (Am. 8:1–6). God was so angry with them that he threatened to send the worst famine possible, "a famine of hearing the words of the Lord" (8:11). As for their religion? "I hate, I despise your religious feasts; I cannot stand your assemblies..." (5:21). Religious devotion without righteousness and justice is a mockery. Only those who "seek me" will "live," declares the Lord (5:4b). There are no short-cuts to divine favor.

I was powerfully reminded of this symbiotic relationship between righteousness and justice in a conversation with a young widow in Kabwe, Zambia. We met when my wife, Kathy, and I were visiting one of our Home-Based Care volunteer groups in an outlying area called Makululu. Her name was Victoria. She had three young children of her own. She was twenty-six years old.

"So why are you here?" I asked. "I mean, you're a widow yourself, yet you're helping other widows."

"They need help," she answered shyly.

"Do you need help too?"

"Yes."

"For your kids?"

"Yes."

"Are they sick?"

"No."

"Are they hungry?"

"Yes."

"So where do you get food?"

Looking away, then slowly upward, she responded quietly, but with strength, "The Lord looks after us."

And, after a long silence, she said, "He is so faithful. I must be too."

"That's why you're here as a volunteer?" I asked.

"Yes."

I was in the presence of a modern-day Job. And Job's wife was present within me. I was from the planet where self-indulgence and individualism ruled. She was from the planet where self-love was abhorrent if it had no counterbalance in love for God and neighbor. She knew *Yahweh Yireh* ("God will provide"). She also knew her neighbor. And she loved both.

Victoria was righteous and just. Living on less than a dollar a day, she was nonetheless fully alive. Adversity had fine-tuned her intuitive knowledge of God and she had hit the sweet spot of the prophetic call. Without theological training she had discovered what one old theologian identified as "the transitive holiness of God."

Holy and Unholy

Before God is anything, he is holy. Spiritually and morally, he is perfect. There is no flaw, no imperfection in him, nor is his holiness ever whimsical or lacking integrity. Eternally he is God, eternally he is holy, eternally he lives apart from his creation, even while he is present everywhere in his love and care.

We, on the other hand, are anything but holy. Spiritually and morally imperfect, we are consistently inconsistent, driven and distracted, dominated by relentless appetites.

For many of us "dysfunction" is our middle name. We spend most of our energies living for ourselves. Captive in space and time we are able, in our best moments, to temporarily approach the outskirts of the heavenlies, but usually we plod about here on earth, our feet not only made of, but weighted down with, great globs of clay. Any connection with God or neighbor seems to be subject to some sort of short-circuit, which presents a problem.

How does our eternal Creator, who "loves us with an everlasting love," relate to us space/timers when we're so unholy? How does "holy" commune with "unholy"? Is there a mechanism, a process, a system? If so, what does it look like? What are its constituent ingredients? How does he "transition" his holiness?

To answer these questions requires another book. But, the two essential ingredients you can guess: they are righteousness and justice.

God has got to do what God has got to do. And he has got to be what he is, not what he's not. He cannot act outside of or beyond his nature. For instance, he cannot lie. He cannot pretend to be what he isn't. He cannot turn a blind eye to sin. He cannot say, "Well, boys will be boys," and let the sinner off the hook without punishing him. His relentless holiness drives everything that he is and does. Yet, even while his holiness requires retribution, his love for us calls for mercy. So, what does he do?

He reveals himself as righteous and just. In righteousness he uncovers his love of holiness; in justice his hatred of sin and its byproducts (broken lives). And as for us, he makes it clear that when we aspire to relate to him, we must embrace the moral expectation of righteousness and accept the judicial consequences of failure. When we look to our neighbor, we must do the same. To be righteous and just, we must fulfill the requirements of relationship with heaven and earth. Otherwise, our Maker must pass us by.

This is more than a touch onerous, we may think; indeed, it appears grossly unfair. God doesn't require these exacting standards of dogs or horses. Why is he picking on us? Because, unlike the rest of creation, we have been created "in His image" (Gen. 1:27). He expects and demands more of us because we're the only ones who are like him. And he intends to see us holy when we reach "the other side." To that end, he insists that we possess the DNA of righteousness and justice in space and time, so that we can truly be "the planting of the Lord" when we see and fellowship with him "face to face."

"Yes, but," we stammer. "We try to be righteous and just, but we never succeed. We don't have what it takes." Like Isaiah we see ourselves as inexpressibly unclean, leprous even. With him we cry, "Woe to me! I am ruined! For I am a man of unclean lips, and I live among a people of unclean lips, and my eyes have seen the King, the Lord Almighty" (6:5). Righteousness is beyond us. Retribution awaits.

But God, who "is rich in mercy," says, "Yes, you are unclean. Yes, you deserve death for your sin. But here's the deal. Let me become sin for you, even though I know no sin. Let me take your punishment for you. Let me become your righteousness." Enter Jesus, the Lamb of God, stage right. Redeemed, we exit, stage left. In Christ we are made new creatures. In him we "live and move and have our being" (Acts. 17:28). Because of him we're able to live the only kind of "religion that God our Father accepts as pure and faultless" (Jas. 1:27). We "look after orphans and widows in their distress" (justice) and "keep [ourselves] from being polluted by the world" (righteousness). In Christ we are declared righteous. Empowered by Christ, we are able to act justly. In Christ, and only in him, we are "perfect ... as [our] heavenly Father is perfect" (Mt. 5:48). Thus, Africa has a Victoria who knows "the Name" and the names of the poor. And, North America has me, who is only beginning to get acquainted with both. That's why I'm praying that I will "grow in the grace and knowledge of our Lord and Savior Jesus Christ" (2 Pet. 3:18).

James, Job, and John Milton

If the righteous are not just, they're not righteous at all. James, Jesus's half-brother, put it well: "What good is it, my brothers, if a man claims to have faith but has no deeds? Can such faith save him? Suppose a brother or sister is without clothes and daily food. If one of you says to him, 'Go, I wish you well; keep warm and well fed,' but does nothing about his physical needs, what good is it? In the same way, faith by itself, if it is not accompanied by action, is dead" (Jas. 2:14–17).

My hero, Job, is a great example of a *zadik* ("a righteous man"). He was a man who "rescued the poor" and the "fatherless," who cared for the "dying," assisted the "blind" and the "lame," and was a "father" or "provider" for the needy. He made "the widows' hearts to sing for joy." He rescued "victims" from the "fangs of the wicked." In summary, he says, "I put on righteousness as my clothing; justice was my robe and my turban" (Job 29:12–17). He was the kind of man who "exalts a nation" (Prov. 14:34). He was righteous both in word and in deed. He practised what he preached.

Job's mantle was justice, or *zadkah* in Hebrew. Here's a second word, *shefet*. Whereas *zadkah* (the noun for *zedek*) has a dual meaning ("righteousness, justice"), *mishpat* (the noun for *shefet*) means basically one thing: justice (although there are nuances of "ordinance, custom, manner"). It is a powerful word, especially when you realize that it describes Israel's messiah's mandate: "I will put my Spirit on him and he will bring justice to the nations" (Isa. 42:1). And the integrity of the Almighty's judgments resonates with unassailable purity. "Will not the Judge of all the earth do right?" ("Will not the 'Shofet' of all the earth do 'mishpat'?" Gen. 18:25). Won't the judge do justice? Of course he will, for he is "elohe mishpat Yahweh," the "God of justice" (Isa. 30:18b). He "loves the just" (Ps. 37:28), or as the New Living Translation puts it, "the Lord loves justice."

Just as justice is an attribute of God, and all true justice (like all true creativity) finds its source in him, we, who have been created "in his image," are to be just in our relationships and in our judicial processes. We are to be just in our speaking, our thinking, and in our doing: "The mouth of the righteous man utters wisdom, and his tongue speaks what is just" (Ps. 37:30); "The plans of the righteous are just..." (Prov. 12:5); "And what does the Lord require of you? To act justly and to love mercy and to walk humbly with your God" (Mic. 6:8). When we act justly and do justice, "it brings joy to the righteous but terror to evildoers" (Prov. 21:15). Justice is more than a byproduct of righteousness, it is what the *zadikim* do, much to the discomfort of the unrighteous. John Milton, that great poet, put it this way: "Truth and justice are all one; for truth is but justice in our knowledge, and justice is but truth in our practice. ... For truth is properly no more than contemplation, and her utmost efficiency is but teaching; but justice in her very essence is all strength and activity, and hath a sword put into her hand to use against all violence and oppression on earth" (John Milton, *Eikonoklastes,* quoted in *Systematic Theology* by A.G. Strong, Judson Press, p. 292). So, when "the alien, the orphan, and the widow" cry for justice, the righteous had better respond, quickly, consistently, and with strength—if there's any justice. Otherwise, all is lost.

Bright Light in a Dark Nation

As I implied in recounting my conversation with Victoria, I see myself as an underachiever regarding righteousness and justice. There's not much "light" in me. Theologically I know that "Christ is our righteousness" and I accept that truth wholeheartedly. But it's the outworking in space and time of that heavenly reality that is my Achilles' heel. If I'm not focused, and intentional in my actions, justice can very easily disappear from my radar screen. And often it's the very people who should be objects of justice who model just behavior. For instance, I'll never forget an amazing example of "light" my wife and I witnessed in central Zimbabwe.

Brutal political repression, drought, and famine had paralyzed the nation. Everywhere we looked we saw long queues for petrol (which is rarely available), for cash (people stand for hours waiting to withdraw a maximum $3 per day), and for bread. Entire communities had been razed by government bulldozers. People slept in the street, under trees, in the parks. And this was just Harare!

Throughout the nation, people were living like stray dogs. I'll never be able to erase the image of several displaced Zimbabwean families living in a church-owned chicken coop in Mutare. And, in central Zimbabwe, people were literally starving to death.

A newly planted church in Harare, of about one hundred people, decided they had to do something about these starving folk. Even though they were small and poor themselves, they felt that their faith required them to reach out to "the least of these, their brethren." As city folk they were heavily burdened with life, but the country people were about to lose theirs, so they connected with a veteran missionary who had access to the Canadian Food Grains Bank. Through a lot of procedural diligence and coordinated effort on the part of several volunteers, they managed to arrange for a major shipment of cornmeal to be sent to the severely afflicted area. Kathy and I were driven for four hours to the country church where the food was to be delivered that day.

As we turned off the main highway onto what was no more than a dirt cart path, our driver (and distribution coordinator) told us there would be 1,000 people coming for food. "In fact they're already here," he said. We looked around and saw no one. "Keep looking," he said.

We were bumping up and down the heavily rutted road as we descended into a valley surrounded by low-lying hills. These kopjes were topped with a Zimbabwean natural wonder: random piles of massive rocks and boulders that look like the artwork of a giant sculptor. There in the shadows of these humongous works, on almost every hill, sat groups of thin, patient people, waiting for the delivery truck to arrive. Seeing us, many broke into huge smiles and waved enthusiastically. But no one ran out of the shadows to our vehicles. Everyone stayed in place.

"They're very disciplined," the driver answered our unasked question. "No food riots here."

"No kidding!" I responded. "We've heard of and seen a few scenes of complete confusion and violence, especially when food arrives among starving people."

"True, but these folk are aware that if there's a food fight, the truck driver may simply leave. And there'll be no more food from Canada."

"So, how have they managed this?" Kathy asked.

"Each group is from a village. Each village has a headman. Each headman has a list of names. If your name is not on the list, you get no food. If you jump the queue, you get no food. No order, no food."

"So what's going to happen?" I asked.

"See that building at the bottom of the valley? That's the church. The truck will arrive soon. When it does, the various groups will come down from the hills in a prearranged order. The headman will read their names one by one, the food will be given, they'll move on, and the next group will do the same. When everyone has their food, the leftover bags will be stored in the church."

"Just like that?"

"Yep."

And that's how it happened. Just like that. The big tractor-trailer lurched over the uneven ground and arrived at the humble church building three hours late (flat tire). There was no rush of humanity from the hills. The truck driver and his assistant climbed up onto the trailer, removed the tarpaulin, then gave the signal to the nearest hill. Slowly but surely, their grim, thin faces near bursting with muted excitement, a line of walking skeletons came down from the kopje. Quietly and in order, they sat on the ground, the headman read their names, they walked over to the truck, strong young men lowered heavy bags of cornmeal to their bony shoulders, and, their faces now wreathed in smiles, they began the slow trek back to their villages. Just like that.

One small group of women, bowed under the weight of this food from heaven, burst into a hymn of thanksgiving as they walked away. "God is so good, he's so good to me!" they sang. I watched them for a long time as they slowly disappeared up into the hills. The music faded with them as they passed from view.

The headman of the headmen, the "chief," came over to me. Knowing that Kathy and I were Canadians, he thanked us for sending the food from 8,700 miles away to their impoverished villages.

"It wasn't us," I replied quickly, "it was the church in Harare who sent it."

"I know, I know," he said, "but if it weren't for you Christians in Canada, we would have no one to turn to."

"Well, it was a joint effort," I said. "We care about you."

"Thank you, man of God," he gripped my hand, his clear eyes moist, "you've saved our lives."

"No, not me," I mumbled, barely able to speak. "It was those dear brothers and sisters of yours in Harare who did this."

"Then I'll take it as from the Lord," he whispered.

"Exactly," I whispered back. "It's from the Lord."

Yahweh Yireh. Right belief, right action. Once again I had to find a private place to weep. I'd been blinded by the light.

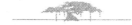

Faithfulness and Unfailing Love

This book is subtitled, "A Christian Response to AIDS in Africa." It might just as easily read, "A Christian Response to the Victims of AIDS in Africa: The Orphans and Widows." But this latter subtitle is a touch too long and ungainly. Nevertheless, the Christian response must be to the orphans and widows. HIV is the enemy; it is creating the greatest wave of orphans and widows in history, but our response must start with the victims, even as we pray for and donate monies to a search for a vaccine to destroy this vile threat. We're in a war, a tiring and eviscerating war. It's hard to keep going. It's tough staying faithful.

Moses had a word for us when we feel like quitting, when our hearts and minds have gone dry with sustained effort, as though we have sweated the very essence of our vision out of our pores. We're disheartened by death, overcome with the sadness that surrounds, beaten down by pursuing justice, broken just like the broken ones we're trying to heal. "Look to the Lord," he says.

> ³Oh, praise the greatness of our God! He is the Rock, his works are perfect, and all his ways are just. A faithful God who does no wrong, upright and just is he. (Deut. 32:3, 4)

"First of all," he says, "remember your foundation." "He is the Rock" on which your life is built. The superstructure may get beaten down sometimes, the walls may need repair, the roof may leak, and a window or two may be cracked and broken, but the foundation is solid! So deal with the "slings and arrows of outrageous fortune," remember that "man is born to trouble as the sparks fly upward," and get on with it. You may be shuddering but you're unshakable, you may be stressed but you're unmovable, you may be flawed but your life is built on the "perfect" and "just" greatness of "our God" the "Rock." He is righteous (*zedek*) and just (*yashar*). And, so important this one—he is faithful.

In Old Testament prophetic passages, faithfulness is often tied to righteousness and justice. Israel's future messiah is described in Isaiah, Chapter 11, as "judging the needy" with "righteousness," and "faithfulness" is the "sash around his waist" (vv. 4, 5). Messiah's mandate, as we've noted previously, is to "bring justice to the nations" (Isa. 42:1), and he'll bring it forth "in faithfulness" (v. 3). In Habbakuk 2:4, we read that the *zadik* (the righteous or the just) "will live by His faithfulness."

In the Hebrew language, the word for faithfulness comes from the root *a-m-n* (*aman*). It has a variety of meanings depending on how it's used. It can mean "to confirm, support, uphold," or it can mean "to be established, to be faithful," and it can also mean "to be certain, to believe in." The noun *omen* (pronounced o-mane) is the word from which the English "amen" is derived. The basic concept of the word is "to be certain" like the certainty we see in the strong arms of a father holding a helpless infant. His strong arms and hands are like pillars of support. The baby can count on them. They'll never fail.

This fail-safe commitment reminds me of Precious, a seventeen-year-old girl we met in Tanzania. Her story is one of the most powerful examples of faithfulness I know. It moves me every time I think of it.

Kathy and I had flown across Lake Victoria that day, from Mwanza to Bukoba. Touching down on a gravel landing strip, we taxied to a little cement-block building where we were met by a local faith-based charity worker in an old four-wheel drive vehicle. From there we drove two-and-a-half hours north, up to where this Tanzanian panhandle meets the Ugandan border. (It's called a panhandle because it is a narrow strip of land bounded by Burundi and Rwanda on the west, Lake Victoria on the east, and Uganda on the north. It is also believed that the panhandle is where HIV first entered Tanzania, from Uganda.)

The going was rough, but the scenery beautiful. As we climbed hills and descended into valleys, we were surrounded by lush banana trees. And, on both sides of the road, there were countless Tanzanians with huge loads of bananas piled on their Chinese-made bicycles heading to markets miles away. We were struck to see a man pushing a sick old woman in a wheelbarrow. "The local ambulance," our driver said with a kind smile, "is taking her to the clinic."

"How far is that?" I asked.

"Oh, maybe a five-hour walk."

Five hours? Up and down those hills? How could he manage? Then again, maybe the old woman was his mother, or a dearly loved aunt, so how could he not? And how would she manage? Those old bones compressed against the confined, jarring sides of the wheelbarrow, her shoulders and neck aching with the strain of keeping her head up, her legs numbed by dangling over the hard edge, the unsuspended frame conveying every bump, every stone, every wobble of the unshod wheel. "There's Job again," I thought. And even though he was taking her across the road and down a footpath to the valley below, I felt a strong urge to lend a hand, to help in some way.

"Maybe that old woman is not as old as she looks. Maybe she has AIDS. Maybe she's his wife," I thought. I looked back, about to say something to our driver, but the ambulance had already disappeared into the dense foliage like a mirage in a desert of human suffering. For the next forty minutes we traveled in silence. Then we reached the end of the road. It was time to get out and walk.

It was a difficult climb up the well-worn path through the banana trees to the village. As we approached, we were soon swarmed with scores of children, laughing, holding our hands (at one point I had three little hands in each of mine), and rubbing our arms (they're not used to seeing hair on anyone's arms). Suddenly the village appeared. There in the lush surroundings of the banana forest were several little *rondavaals* (mud-walled, thatched-roofed huts). In the excitement of our arrival, it took a few minutes before it hit us. Kathy and I looked at each other and asked the same question at the same time, "Where are the adults?"

There were none. They had all died from AIDS. This was an orphan village, one of scores in rural Africa. A community of children raising themselves.

Our host had arranged for us to meet Precious. At age seventeen, she was one of the elders in the village. She took us to her *rondavaal* where she and her brother and sister lived. Ducking our heads we entered through the tiny door into a round, bare room carpeted in sweet grass. There, against the wall on the far side her brother and sister sat, their eyes large and their expressions a mix of fear and intrigue. We sat on the floor opposite, and Precious began to tell her story.

Five years ago, when she was twelve, her father became very sick. For two years she and her mother cared for him as he slowly wasted away. They knew he was dying of AIDS, but like most other afflicted families in Africa, they feared the stigma and discrimination associated with "the slim disease." So they said he was sick with "pneumonia, kidney infection, boils, diarrhea," or whatever opportunistic infection happened to be wreaking havoc with his weakened immune system at the time. When Precious was fourteen her father died.

Even as they laid his emaciated body to rest, Precious was aware that her mother had taken ill. For the next two years she cared for her dying mother. When she was sixteen, Precious buried her. Now she shifted her full-time care to her brother and sister. An orphan herself, she had sole responsibility for two other orphans. Her situation seemed beyond hope.

Fortunately, she found a job as a domestic for a small business. It was a two-and-a-half hour walk away. So every morning Precious got up at three-thirty and left at four to be at work for six-thirty. She put in an eight-hour day, then walked two-and-a-half hours back. There she was, a small teenaged Tanzanian girl, walking five hours every day, by herself, in the dark. Six days a week.

For this she earns $60 a year. With that income she's able to buy three outfits a year of used clothes for herself and her two siblings (yes, they wear the same clothes every day), and she's able to feed them two meals of ground corn a day. And, most important, she's also able to pay school fees for her brother and sister.

"I have a dream," she said with quiet confidence. "I want my brother and sister to become schoolteachers. I want them to have respect, and to be able to care for themselves one day."

There's no money for anything else. No medicines. No lock on the flimsy door to protect them from drunken raids on the village by predatory males. No father. No defender.

"Do you go to church?" Kathy asked.

"Oh, yes, ma'am, every Sunday. We love Jesus. He cares for us."

At this point I had to go outside to gather myself. Here was a young woman laying down her life for someone else. She knew that by the time her siblings were teachers she would be too old for marriage, illiterate, and of use to no one. Yet she got up in the middle of the night and walked alone in the darkness to see a dream come true that in the end would factor her out. If ever I'd seen someone whose life was an active illustration of righteousness and justice, she was that person. And such staggering faithfulness!

Faithfulness essentially is "showing up for work." There's nothing romantic or appealing about it; you just grind it out, day after day, year after year. But, like building a building brick by brick, if you keep at it, you will eventually have constructed something that will last. You build a marriage that way. You build a career that way. You build a life that way. Precious is building Tanzania that way.

The prophet Hosea, no slouch himself when it came to faithfulness, said:

> *Sow for yourselves righteousness, reap the fruit of unfailing love, and break up your unplowed ground; for it is time to seek the Lord, until he comes and showers righteousness on you. (Hos. 10:12)*

Righteousness in this passage is seen as seed, fruit, and rain. You sow it, you reap it, and it irrigates your soul. But, before any of this happens, you've got to "break up your unplowed ground." We've all got hardened places in our lives that must be aggressively plowed into if there's any hope of rain penetrating, seed germinating, and a harvest gathered. And it's going to take committed, consistent effort. There will be no justice, no righteousness, no hope for orphan or widow without "unfailing love," the love of a Precious.

Journal
Esther's Hymn of Salvation

A wildebeest cow is giving birth. She's chosen a spot in the middle of the grazing herd. This is the most vulnerable she's been to a lion attack since she herself was born. She instinctively seeks the protection of the others.

Stoically she stands, seeking no assistance, an occasional grunt the only sign of effort, the emerging calf slowly sliding from the birth canal. The newborn is about halfway out when it happens. The zebras on the fringe give a warning cry and like a shot the herd is off, running madly from the attacking lions. The birthing mother instinctively runs too, the calf dangling from her hindquarters. But she runs slowly, awkwardly, and the lions, fine-tuned to single out the sick, the aged, and the lame, zero in. In a flash they're on her. Heroically she gives a final push, the calf falls to the ground, and she carries the three lions on her back several yards before her knees buckle. She dies quickly, the lions gorging on her flesh even as she breathes her last.

Amazingly they ignore the helpless calf who, oblivious to the danger, is trying to stand. After several attempts he finally succeeds, wobbling on his spindly legs as if he is a sapling blowing in the wind. The lions continue to ignore him, but he's not out of danger. As certain as night follows day, the sights and sounds of a lion kill attract other predators, all surrounding the scene in a distinct pecking order. First the hyenas, then the jackals, and finally the vultures—all expert at reducing a carcass to bone. They keep their distance from the lions and from each other. They're competitors, but they respect the capability of the other and the vulnerability of self in ascending order.

The calf wobbles, falls, rights himself, and bleats. Every competing predator sees, but he's too close to the feeding lions for anyone to risk taking him. The closest hyena, the leader of the pack, inches closer. She has had many close encounters in the past with her mortal enemies, and bears the battle scars. She's cagey, experienced, and brazenly courageous. Suddenly she dashes from the long grass, swoops in, takes the calf by the neck, and runs wildly away before the distracted lions can respond. In a few minutes the calf has been devoured. The symbiotic relationship of predator and prey has performed its one-act drama on the stage of the savanna once again. And, as always, Mother Nature has favored the strong. The weak have no defense.

When Glory Mbene was born, her mother, Esther, gave birth beneath a thorn tree on the outskirts of her village. She was all alone. Fourteen years of age, the youngest wife of four to the village headman, she was used to bearing the scorn of the older wives, doing the grunt work, and expecting no help, affirmation, or love from any of them, including her forty-year-old "husband." Rather, the order of her life was rife with physical, verbal, and sexual abuse, where "relationship" was equivalent to "pain." She suffered silently, and valued what few moments she had to herself like gold. Fourteen going on forty, she was a survivor.

Esther wasn't sure who the father was. Her husband gave her to male visitors on a regular basis. She hated it when an "uncle" came for an overnight visit. As the men went through the expected hospitality protocols—handshaking, smiles, pleasantries, tea, conversation, more tea—it was she who was required to fill the visitor's cup, and as she did so, her head bowed in deference, serving the tea on her knees, she could feel his eyes consuming her, his tone smug and lustful. He knew she was his for the night, his to do whatever he demanded. She always felt unclean after these violations. Unclean, sometimes for days. Maybe forever.

As a wife of the headman she was free of common rape. No man or boy in the village wanted to mess with his property. But other girls were fair game. Esther's closest friend, Hope, had been brutally raped by four teenaged boys on her daily walk for water (she spent six hours a day going to and from the bore hole). After their foul work was done, they had ran away, leaving her almost lifeless on the ground. A nine-year-old boy, witness to the scene, had crept up to her inert figure and mimicked the teenagers, mounting her ineptly, injuring her further, and had then scampered off. At a distance he picked up a rock and threw it, hitting her on her bare back, cracking a rib. She lay there all night, crawling home the next morning, where her father beat her for her absence. Later, as she slowly recovered, she said to Esther, "They treat the dog better than they treat me. I wish I were dead." In some ways she and most of the women in Africa were dead. They might be walking and breathing, but they had no freedom, no rights, no respect. One could say they were the walking dead, zombie-like creatures with no usefulness other than drawing water, hewing wood, and servicing sexual predators.

About a year ago Esther had noticed a distinct decline in the health of her husband and his first two wives. All three of them seemed to be more vulnerable than others to colds, fevers, and nagging muscle and joint pain. Colds seemed to drag on forever, sometimes leading to weeks of pneumonia with racking coughs and bloody phlegm. Lately her husband had developed skin sores that wouldn't go away. He had lost weight, and he'd become listless and distant. All of this sickness in the household increased the burden Esther had to bear. Her days were spent fetching water, cleaning sores, changing befouled bedclothes, cooking food, and bearing the berating of the third wife, who, at this point, was as healthy as Esther. Even as her body began to swell with new life, Esther was required to work from early morning to late at night. Who cared if she was pregnant? She was the household's beast of burden and she'd better get to it or there would be hell to pay.

Now, as she labored through agonizing contractions beneath the thorn tree, the three at home were totally invalid, bedridden, and dying. The words of the third wife, who had been losing weight herself lately, screeched like fingernails on a blackboard: "Get out! Have your brat, and get back! You're the reason we're all sick. You've put a curse on us!" She punched Esther in the stomach as she left, "Have another witch, 'Witch!'" And she screamed at Esther's retreat: "I'm going to the Healer! He'll make me well, and then we'll deal with you." The "healer" was the local witch doctor. Esther would return to the best counter-curse her accuser could buy.

Indeed, the next few years were like a curse. Esther slaved in her dying household in conditions that only the oppressed of history can appreciate. She wasn't just "paying," she was living in hell. Six months after Glory's birth, her husband and wife number one died. Esther was shunned at the funeral, and more counter-curses were brought against her. Wives numbers two and three, both bedridden, were relentless in their demands, and, to make matters much worse, her departed husband's mother had come to live with them. Tempestuous and given to blood-curdling rages, she forced Esther to build her own small hut and live next to the latrine. There, in exile, with the stench of the toilet her constant companion, Esther raised Glory and three more infants that had been brought to her for care—they were all children of extended family members who had died from "the slim disease." She may have been seen as a witch, but Esther had voluminous breasts for nursing and a seemingly tireless back. Beaten and downtrodden, she refused to give up on life. Unlike her friend Hope, she had hope.

The only freedom allowed her was attendance at a rural church on Sundays, an early morning hour's walk away. Unlike her family and neighbors, Esther was a follower of Jesus. Held in the grip of animistic superstition and fear, her family projected their bondage onto Esther, but she was able to suffer tirelessly because she saw herself under the protection of the great sufferer himself, Israel's messiah, who was "despised and rejected of men, a man of sorrows, and acquainted with grief." She found great solace in her savior's acquaintance with human misery. He had endured it, and risen above it. She would, too. Like Job, she knew "that my redeemer liveth." Her faith gave her a backbone of steel and a heart of flesh. She cared for the orphans imposed upon her like she cared for Glory herself. She had a bottomless capacity to love. And, she could sing like an angel.

Her faith was severely tested on Glory's first birthday. Wife number three died, and even before the body was cold, Esther's mother-in-law banished her from the property. So there she was, a fifteen-year-old widow, caring for four orphans, with nowhere to go and no one to support her.

Her first night of banishment found her and her four children sleeping under the very thorn tree where she had given birth to Glory. On the way there she had found a wheelbarrow that seemed ownerless, and in her desperation, had loaded her babies and some paltry supplies on it, and had pushed it to the thorn tree, praying that she would be spared a violent visit from someone claiming it as his own. Early the next morning she pushed the wheelbarrow with its precious cargo three hours to the bore hole, hoping to connect with a woman there who also attended her church. To her great relief ("Praise the Lord!") the friends met, and her kind fellow-pilgrim arranged temporary housing for her while she gathered the "supplies" necessary to build her own shelter—stray pieces of lumber, plastic sheeting, corrugated fiberglass "roofing," and whatever else could be used in the construction. Two days later she moved in, thrilled that she'd been given a cooking pot, a kettle, and a discarded back seat from an abandoned car for a bed.

There she set up house. There she cared for her four orphan babies. There she waited for her "redeemer" to supply her needs "according to his riches in glory." And it was there her redeemer did so by providing a humble, poor, but caring local church to be a father to her fatherless children, and a defender of her vulnerable household. She truly saw the Almighty as a constant presence, a loving father, a protecting husband. She meant it every time she "testified" on Sundays at the church service: "My God has supplied all my needs. He is faithful, loving, and kind. As for me and my household, we will serve the Lord." She testified and lived with the conviction of someone who knew whom and what she believed.

She sang that way, too. When I first met her, she sang a solo at church. I was the visiting preacher, the mzungu, from faraway Canada, the "man of God" who was to be revered and respected. As I heard Esther sing, I was bowled over by the power of her presence and the clarity of her message. She sang a Western hymn in my honor. As it so happened, it was (and is) one of my all-time favorites. The lyrics are timeless and true. But in Esther's voice, and with Esther's integrity, the words shone out like light in the darkness:

> Great is thy faithfulness,
> O God my father,
> There is no shadow of turning
> With thee.
> Thou changest not,
> Thy compassions they fail not,
> As thou hast been,
> Thou forever wilt be...

I wept shamelessly. Once again I was a student in the presence of a master. She was only a third my age, but Esther stood before me a true "citizen of the kingdom," someone who knew what she was singing about. Someone who could show the way. As she sang, I felt her soul reaching out to mine: "Come, Pasta, come with me, let me show you the land that is fairer than day."

Chapter 2
HIV/AIDS:
Killing the Young

*I*n this chapter I'm going to "bear witness." It's not a happy story, but I feel compelled by what I've seen to share it with as many people as possible. Before I do, however, I need to tell you how I became a witness in the first place.

It started in Jerusalem. Kathy and I had been invited by Israeli government officials (from the ministries of Tourism, Religion, and Foreign Affairs) to start a nondenominational church in 1981. This was an offer we couldn't refuse. (The story of how all that came about is a book in itself.) We established the church (now known as the King of Kings Assembly, with offices and auditorium in the Clal Center at Davidka Square), and soon people from all over the world began dropping in. One Sunday night, in 1984, a pastor from South Africa attended our service. Afterwards he introduced himself and asked if I would be interested in speaking at a major pastors' conference the following year in his country. Of course I said yes.

Thus began a long-term relationship with South Africa and hundreds of South African pastors. In fact, one of those pastors came to Jerusalem and worked on our staff for three years before returning to Durban to establish a church. Years later he would play a key role in our story.

After seven years in Jerusalem I had cultivated a leadership team that was more capable than I. Indeed, I had worked myself out of a job. I was pleased to hand over the church to this terrific team and move back to North America. For eight years Kathy and I were involved in national television work. Then we took a hiatus from television and moved to Vancouver to pastor a church. It was while we were there that our pastor friend from Durban called. He wanted us to come to South Africa and spend a few weeks with him, his church, and his leaders. So, in August 1999 we flew to Durban.

One night Kathy and I were watching the South African television news. The news reader, as calmly as if she were reading the weather forecast, read this: "The South African government have just released a report indicating that life expectancy in our nation has gone down ten years because of HIV/AIDS." I was shocked. I checked with Kathy to see if I had heard the report accurately. "That's what I heard," she said. I felt like I'd been kicked in the stomach. I hardly slept that night.

The next morning I "crashed" a small meeting of church leaders in Durban. I got right to the point. "Fellas," I said to somewhat startled preachers around the table, "what are you doing about HIV/AIDS?"

There was silence. Then one of them said, "Nothing, Jim." He shrugged. "We know we should be doing something. But we're not..." He looked away.

What I said next I had never said, thought, or read before. It came out of left field, as they say. It blind-sided me.

"Pastors, every church in South Africa has got to become a Mother Teresa. If that little Albanian nun could impact the whole world by ministering to the dying in the streets of Calcutta, what could the thousands of churches in South Africa do with this death culture that's descending on your nation? What's more, there's four things you've got to emphasize. First, you've got to have a major HIV/AIDS awareness campaign so that your people turn from denial and face the reality of HIV/AIDS as a church issue. Second, you're going to need a comprehensive HIV/AIDS educational approach, especially for the children in your churches who are twelve years of age and younger. Third, you must develop a vast care and housing infrastructure for children orphaned by AIDS. And last, you need to create an army of thousands of volunteers providing home-based palliative care to those dying of AIDS."

No one spoke. I myself had nothing further to say. It was as if I'd fired all the shells in my gun and what remained was a whisper of smoke and ringing in my ears. I was surprised at what I had just said, even embarrassed, for I was aware that I had intruded upon their space. I'd come unannounced and uninvited. Who did I think I was?

I smiled weakly, mumbling something about flying back to North America that evening, said goodbye, and left. Thirty-six hours later we were in Atlanta. South Africa seemed another place in the solar system. And, as we landed in Vancouver, it was as if my harangue to the preachers hadn't happened. I quickly became absorbed in my work.

Two months later an e-mail arrived. "We can't get away from the vision you've cast," it said. "We've called a broader meeting for South African pastors in January 2000. We meet in Johannesburg. Can you attend and restate your vision?" I quickly responded, "I'm there." Over the next two months I resigned from the church, and Kathy and I founded a federal charity that would enable us to operate internationally in social justice work. January 9, 2000, was our last Sunday in Vancouver. Two weeks later I was in Johannesburg.

All of this, of course, was not as easy as it sounds. The resignation from the church precipitated a "dark night of the soul" in my life. Here I was, pastoring a large church with 2,500 people on the rolls, only two and a half years into it, and now I was resigning? Leaving a fixed income, a fixed address, and the "status" of pastoring one of Vancouver's largest churches, for what? An idea? A vision? How to pay the bills? Where to live? Was I prepared to live indefinitely with no fixed address and no fixed income? What about the people? Wasn't I letting them down? What about Kathy? What about HIV/AIDS? I was no medical expert, nor was the church here or there interested in hearing about something associated with dubious sexual practices. One of my very best friends, upon hearing what I was proposing to do, looked at me in disbelief and said, "Jimmy, nobody cares about HIV/AIDS. No one will listen. No one will support you. I think you need to rethink." And besides, I didn't know I'd "cast a vision" anyway. I'd just opened my mouth and those words came out. Maybe this road less traveled was nothing but a quixotic goose chase. And yet...

My life had been predicated on heaven's word to me now, present tense, relevant, current, the "Shepherd's voice," if you will, telling me which way to go. I've always had a high view of scripture (as you can undoubtedly tell), but that high view saw more than history, integrity, and revelation; it saw a God, not limited by space and time, everlastingly present, eternally current, speaking to his people today with as much power and compelling love as yesterday.

I felt in the grip of an irresistible call to live on the keen knife-edge of what would become the greatest threat to mankind in history. At the heart of it was God's heart for the orphan and widow. What would come of it only God knew. But somehow I had heard the "voice" and my response echoed the words of God-fearing souls throughout the ages who, upon encountering the brooding, intimidating, and compelling presence, found themselves without prior notice or conscious preparation saying, "Here am I. Send me."

One of the South African pastors met me at the airport and we drove to Pretoria where I was booked to stay at a severe, barracks-style hostel. A few other foreign pastors were already booked in. I threw my bag onto the empty cot, said hello to the ubiquitous gecko on the wall, and opened the window onto the adjacent Pretoria zoo whose perimeter was a mere 10 feet from where I stood. I was jetlagged, dislocated, and felt so out of place. I could hear the other pastors out in the hall, one on his cellphone, another click-clacking his way over the keyboard of a laptop, friendly conversation and laughter filling the air, and I thought, "All those guys have jobs. Income. Offices. Secretaries. Homes. I've lost all that. I'm adrift." And I felt tremors of panic deep down in my chest. "Get a grip, Jim. Get a grip. You'll be okay. Don't bolt now. Keep going." It took forever to get to sleep. When I did it was to the soothing sounds of lions aspirating 30 feet away, their deep-chested rumblings resonating with the throbbing of my troubled heart.

The next morning we drove to a church in Johannesburg where the meeting was to take place. The men were nice enough as we exchanged pleasantries over coffee, but it seemed to me that they were all nonverbally saying, "And why are we here? And what do you, a White North American, have to say to us?" I felt like a doctoral student about to face his inquisitors at the oral defense of his thesis. The meeting was called to order, and the chairman, after some preliminary remarks about the scourge of AIDS and comments about our ad hoc meeting in Durban, said, "So now, Jim, will you please restate your vision about how our churches can address the issue?"

The first time in Durban I had blurted this "vision" out, without forethought. This time I'd had months to get ready. I've spoken publicly over 4,000 times in my life and can't say I've ever really been nervous, but now I felt fear and trepidation like I'd never known. It took all I had to restate the vision in a level voice. When I finished, a young pastor of two churches in Soweto leaped to his feet and shouted, "Yes! Yes! This is the vision for our nation!" Then everyone started talking at once. Finally the chairman called for silence and said, "Jim, it appears that we want to adopt your vision. And we will, if you will show us the way." I was speechless. What did I know? I had no more idea of "the way" than I had of the best route to the South Pole. I felt like Frodo in *The Lord of the Rings*, when the elders of Rivendell were all talking at once, agitated and confused as to what to do with the ring of power. In the midst of the bedlam, he lifted his little voice and said, "I will take the ring, though I do not know the way." I'd already taken several leaps in the dark. Why not another? So, drawing a deep breath, I said quietly, "God helping me, I'll do my best." As they gathered around to pray for me, I gulped back the tears and silently prayed, "Father, show me the way." But I knew from past experience that the Lord had never shown me the way. He had simply been the way. His words were his actions. And all I had to do was act on his word and walk in his shadow.

Within days I was getting e-mails and phone calls from Zambia, Zimbabwe, Malawi, Mozambique, and Tanzania. "Please, Jim, come and do with us what you're doing in South Africa." Kindly, but directly, I e-mailed back: "But I'm not doing anything. Yet. Give me time. Right now all I've got is an idea." And what was that idea? That vision? "Every church a Mother Teresa." I saw a huge delivery mechanism in the massive network of local churches in Africa. A delivery system that, if mobilized, could be the most sustainable and potent enemy of AIDS on the planet. We simply had to engage it. One church at a time.

When we started in 2000, the estimate of deaths due to AIDS each day was approximately 6,000. And, every day, 12,000 young people were newly infected. Every day. By 2002 the UN estimated that about 3 million people had died from AIDS and 5 million had been newly infected. It was about that time that the estimate worldwide for HIV infections topped the 40 million mark—with 30 million of those in sub-Saharan Africa. The growth is exponential. By the year 2020, it is possible that as many as 100 million people will have lost their lives to AIDS. And some experts predict that if current rates of infection continue unchecked, there will be 1 billion people HIV positive by the year 2050. At the time of writing, over 9,000 people a day are dying of AIDS. It's as though twenty-three fully loaded Boeing 747s were to crash. Every day. We've never seen anything like this in history. A whole generation of young people is being wiped out. We're being sucked into the vortex of a demographic black hole. The world, our fragile craft, is slowly but surely being swamped in an unsettled sea of sorrow.

So, the meeting is over. I've committed myself to "carrying the ring." What now? Where do I go from here? The first job was to deal with my ignorance about HIV/AIDS. In the process I needed a crash course in African culture. That's why Kathy and I decided to start in Kwazulu Natal.

Before getting into the story, however, I need to say something about statistics. The main source for HIV/AIDS statistics in Africa is data gathered at neonatal clinics. There are studies done, of course, that go beyond pregnant mothers, but in the main the neonatal statistics provide the backbone of most information that you can glean from magazine articles, newspapers, television reports, and the Internet. This means that the overview we get from such sources is limited and conservative. Kathy and I quickly discovered on our flight from ignorance that there was a great gulf between the "official" statistics and the "anecdotal" estimates we heard from doctors, nurses, clergy, social workers, and various nongovernmental organizations (NGOs). I'm not suggesting that one source is better than the other. I'm simply reporting that it is difficult to get an "accurate" overview. There is one thing certain about HIV/AIDS statistics—they are out of date. The exponential growth of the pandemic is always way ahead of those studying its impact. So, take any statistical description in this book or anywhere else as yesterday's news.

Kwazulu Natal is a province in South Africa located in the so-called coastal strip between Swaziland in the north and East London in the south. Durban is its main urban center. And, according to both official and unofficial sources, it has the highest per-capita rate of HIV infection in the nation. The official sources say South Africa's HIV rate is approximately 21 percent; Kwazulu Natal's is in the 30 percent range.

Several medical professionals in Durban have told us that 40 percent to 60 percent of the patients in their hospitals are there due to HIV-related afflictions. At least a third of the victims are young women between the ages of fifteen and thirty. In many ways, Kwazulu Natal is a microcosm both of South Africa and the rest of sub-Saharan Africa.

Kathy and I started in Durban by participating in a consultation with various experts concerned about the rampant spread of HIV in Kwazulu Natal. We were the only foreigners in the group. They had invited us not because of any expertise we had, but because they had heard of our vision for a massive delivery mechanism of mobilized local churches throughout their land. They wanted to hear our ideas on this, and then let us know what we were up against. So, we did what they asked of us, but we mainly kept our mouths shut and our ears open. In the group were a few doctors, a couple of university professors, some nurses, and several NGO leaders, all of whom were involved directly with the pandemic. They were rich in experience and full of compassion. They both knew and felt what they were talking about.

They told us that the HIV virus was a relative newcomer to South Africa. They had known of its existence since the early 1980s. Now, in early 2000, they had only about fifteen years of data to work with, and were still in the initial stages of trying to understand the rapid spread of the virus. They had, however, some very insightful thoughts and observations.

First of all, on the macro level, they observed that HIV made its entrance on the national stage just as apartheid was in its death throes. The national consciousness was focused on the mounting international pressure on the South African government to end apartheid and release Nelson Mandela from prison. In the latter half of the eighties, South Africa was beginning to convulse with major social and political change. There was talk of open riots in the streets, of an out-of-control revolution, of blood flowing freely as the various political groups fought to fill the impending political vacuum left behind by the old order. Then, to everyone's surprise (and relief), President F.W. de Klerk released Mandela in 1990 and began the final stages of dismantling apartheid. By 1991 a new constitution was in the works, and a few years later Nelson Mandela was South Africa's first Black president. And it all took place peacefully.

The next several years saw South Africa reinventing itself. National attention was focused on peaceful transition and social reconstruction. South Africans basked in newfound international acceptance. Nelson Mandela toured the world with rock-star status. South African athletes were invited back to international matches. Tourism exploded. All was well, and the future was oh so bright—or so it seemed.

Lost in the excitement and glamor of the new era, a new virus relentlessly replicated itself. Transmitted sexually it found a fecund petrie dish in a culture that had been fractured and fragmented by over forty years of apartheid. An entire generation had grown up not knowing their migrant fathers. Separate "homelands" had forced men to work hundreds of miles from home in the mines or on the vast sugar farms of the well-to-do. For months at a time these men lived apart from their wives and children, their sexual needs met by sex workers. Some of them had two families—the one back home and another close to their work. Others simply slept around. There were always willing women, poverty driving them to sell themselves and/or their daughters for money. They didn't see themselves as sex workers; rather, they were merely transacting for bread money. They called it "transactional sex." HIV, being no respecter of nomenclature, simply thrived. Sex is sex, and HIV prospers when sex partners are many and inhibitions few. You might say HIV planted its roots deep in the rich gold mines of South Africa. Even as the gleaming precious metal was brought from the depths, a silent assassin slowly but inexorably emerged from the shadows. A death culture was about to undermine the wealthiest country on the continent.

At the time of our meeting (March 2000) the critical mass of the world's HIV victims was already in South Africa—4.2 million infected (by 2003 that number had grown to 4.3 million, or 21.5 percent of South Africa's 44 million people). They told us that other African countries such as Swaziland, Botswana, and Zimbabwe had higher prevalence rates, but their populations were not large enough to compete with the volume of infected people in South Africa. They acknowledged, however, with a somber tone, that the spread of HIV in these countries to the north had a lot to do with South Africa's truckers, transporting goods and having sex along the way. Indeed, they referred to new studies demonstrating that the dissemination of HIV could be tracked by tracing the highways leading from South Africa to other nations. These roads were like arteries carrying infected blood. It was (and is) a common sight to see women, sometimes with their daughters, flagging truckers down along the highways, or flocking around at petrol stations and truck stops. I myself, a few months after this meeting, was approached at a petrol station in Zambia by a thin little girl in a tattered flower-print dress, "Sex, meester? Sex?" Turning kindly away I saw her haggard mother watching us furtively from the shadows of a roadside kiosk. It tore my heart.

The highway system in South Africa is world class. The quality of the paving, the width of the roads, the maintenance, the accessibility to any point in the nation, are better than many Western nations can boast. But, ironically, these highways are a problem. Mobility is of the highest order, making for a highly mobile population. Not everyone can afford cars, but everyone can afford public transportation. Thus, South Africans move about the nation with alacrity. And, so does HIV. It goes where the people go, which means everywhere.

Cities, of course, are totally accessible, with more and more of South Africa's youth migrating to them. There they become the urban poor, living in irregular settlements (the politically correct term for squatter camps) on the outskirts of the cities. These settlements can be massive. Comprised of shacks constructed from whatever material can be found, fetid with open sewers, maze-like with alleyways and corridors of mud brick, thick with the sounds and smells of compressed humanity, they can stretch for miles and miles around a city.

Khayalitsa comes to mind. Here you have a seemingly unending swath of poverty wrapping itself around much of Cape Town. It gapes like a putrefied wound between this gloriously beautiful city and the pristine Old World elegance of Stellenbosch to the north. Even as the well-heeled residents of these cities enjoy the pleasures of the best of Africa, the urban poor silently, facelessly, passively live their days supported by domestic work, or day-laborer wages several hours' walk another world away. But they're quick to tell you they would rather live this way than dwell in the country. At least they have hope of a job. Make some money. Meet some people. Live a little.

When you fly over these cities you see these irregular settlements in a different light. From 20,000 or 30,000 feet up, they look like rings around a bathtub, or concentric deposits of minerals surrounding a lake that is drying up. I've sometimes wondered if what I'm seeing is a microcosm of our world. Privilege and entitlement stubbornly persist, but increasingly are encircled by billions of impoverished people living on less than a dollar a day. Or, to put it another way, concentrated power at the center dissipates in the concentric detritus of the disempowered. This is not just South Africa's reality, it's our reality. We're all implicated. Rather than look at the mote in their eye, we'd do well to look at the log in our own.

Migration, multiple sex partners, mobility, and urbanization were just some of the markers our friends in Durban underscored as they tried to help us understand the rampant spread of HIV in their country. There were more markers to come. None would be more telling than poverty.

Over coffee, one of the participants told me about something that had just happened in the impoverished Limpopo province. A seventeen-year-old youth had slit his brother's throat to spare him the suffering of starvation and then had plunged the knife into his own chest. They had been living for months with a dying mother who, in despair, had left them, trying to locate her neglectful husband in the mines. It had been weeks since she'd left. They didn't know if she was alive or dead. They were out of food. No one would help them. Desperate, the young man took drastic measures. His brother died. He lived. And now he had been charged with murder. Why? Because his brain and judgment had been clouded by starvation. His heart was broken for his brother. He obviously was depressed, with nowhere to turn, so he took up the knife. As relentless as the force of gravity, poverty claimed another victim.

Poverty is a powerful predator. Think of what it can do. You're a young mother of thirteen years of age. From the day you were able to carry a load on your head, you've been working. You're illiterate, unskilled, and both your parents have died of AIDS. You try to care for your little brother and sister, but it's so hard buying food with the few cents a day your Grannie gives you from her meager pension. Three of your "uncles" expect you to "service" them whenever they show up, drunken and violent. If you're having your period, they beat you.

Last year, at age twelve, you had a baby. He's sick most of the time. Now he has malaria and he's so hot. Nothing will console him. You have no medicine. Your stomach hurts from hunger. One of your uncles just brought a "friend," who raped you. You're bleeding. Your baby is moaning. You just want to die. You wish he would die because at least then he would stop his moaning. Your Grannie is yelling at you to go to the well and get some water—it's a two-hour walk, and the pail is heavy. Last week some boys knocked it over, spilling all the water, and then they raped you, all four of them. Your baby is yelling with pain. You pick up the pail, you strap the baby on your back, you begin the long walk, and then you remember the smelly "long-drop" toilet on the way. You return home several hours later with water, but without a son. He lies dying at the bottom of a filthy hole.

He didn't die, however. Someone heard his cry and rescued him. A local charity was notified and he was brought to a humble, under-funded hospice. He's very sick. In fact he has just had a stroke. His left arm is curled up to his chest and the left side of his face is lifeless. The nurse suspects he has lost his hearing as well, "They often do, you know," she tells me. "Sometimes they go blind too."

"From a stroke?" I ask dumbly.

"Yes, pastor, from a stroke."

I hold his little body in my arms and am overwhelmed. The next day he breathes his last and leaves this too cruel world. We never knew his name.

Poverty pushes you into the ground. It compresses you. It reduces you to something subhuman. It makes you powerless, then mocks your powerlessness by "subletting" your victimhood. Disease gets you. Predatory males exploit you. Neighbors steal from you. Dirt, dust, rats, and malarial mosquitoes afflict you. But worst of all, hope for a future dies a lingering death. Your eyes glaze, and you look like the walking dead. And in so many ways you are. It's not as if this thing is going to pass. It's not like the flu, or a phase in your life that will eventually give way. No. This is how you live. This is how you are. This is how it will be for the rest of your life. It's a blessing to die young.

Yes, this is the reality for millions of Africans, especially the women. Another participant in the Durban meeting told us about her organization's work with widows.

"Apart from the well-educated and wealthy women, who are few," she said, "life for most women is terrible. Widows have it even worse."

"How so?" asked Kathy.

"Let me tell you about a widow we're working with just outside of Pietermaritzburg," she replied.

"She has four children, the oldest ten, the youngest two, and she's four months pregnant."

"How old is she?" I asked.

"Twenty-four. Her husband died two months ago from AIDS. Right after the funeral her husband's family swooped in and took everything, then kicked her out on the street."

"Took everything?"

"Yes. Her house, her furniture, her kitchen utensils, even her sewing machine. She made a living sewing, you know."

"How could they do that? Didn't she have documents showing ownership of her home at least?"

"No, she didn't. There was a document, but it was in her husband's name. Thus, her in-laws claimed ownership because he belonged to them."

"And she doesn't?"

"No. As far as they're concerned, she died when her husband died. She's garbage."

"What about the kids? What about her pregnancy?"

"They don't care. Takes too much money to raise four kids."

"So what are her options?" Kathy asked. "Can she remarry? Is there any social assistance available? Can the church help her?"

"Only sometimes. And, how I wish. How I wish. This is why we're so excited about your vision."

"Why can't she remarry?"

"Well, technically she could. But who would want her? She's got four kids. One on the way. And she may have HIV. Besides, sex is everywhere for men. So who needs the hassle, the baggage?"

"What about social assistance?"

"There is a little. The government does have some modest, very modest, programs in effect, but generally a widow like her falls through the cracks. She even has little chance of accessing public health care. She's a non-person, with no one to fight for her."

"And the Church?"

"First of all, you need to know that when it comes to HIV, the Church is in denial. They see it as evidence of sexual sin and feel no responsibility for those who are merely reaping what they've sown."

"But surely, HIV is not the issue in her case? It was her husband, not she, who was infected."

"True, but, the Church, like the society, tends to blame the woman for HIV, not the man. And then there's the issue of her pregnancy. Her husband died two months ago. She's four months' pregnant. He was too sick, obviously, to have fathered this one, so she must have been sleeping with someone else."

"But everyone knows most African women can't say no to sex. Any neighbor, brother-in-law, father-in-law, even grandfather could have impregnated her."

"True. But the Church won't acknowledge these possibilities. As far as they're concerned, she's damaged goods. Needs to be avoided, even shunned."

"In Jesus' name, of course," I muttered.

"Sometimes," she continued, "the husband's family will take the widow in, but it's a horrible life."

"Why?"

"She's treated like a slave. Gets all the menial work. Is subject to sexual abuse, and the verbal abuse of a tyrannical mother-in-law. Her life is hell."

"All because she's a woman," Kathy said darkly.

"All because she's a woman."

We were to personally witness over the next few years the gut-wrenching truth of what this woman told us. The status of women is a major subset of the HIV/AIDS pandemic. It's the women who are bearing the brunt. Why, even the pandemic itself seems to discriminate against them—fully two-thirds of the thousands of new infections every day are among young women and girls. Culture and biology conspire against them. Physically, women have far more surface area exposed to the virus in the act of sex than men do. If there is any violence or sexually transmitted infection (STI) creating tears or lesions, the transfer of the virus, I'm told, is pretty much immediate. Studies on men are ongoing, but it is suspected that the portal of entry for HIV is the underside of the foreskin. Circumcised men seem to be much less likely to become infected unless there is an STI present. But, when they are infected, they become death on the prowl for any unfortunate girl who happens to cross their path at the wrong moment. Violent sex is sure to tear the delicate tissues of the female victim. "Dry sex" does it every time. "Dry sex?" you ask. Yes, it has become popular with men in some areas to insist that their women use a powder to dry their natural vaginal fluids to create more sensation. So the men have their "dry" fun, and the women are taken one step closer to the grave.

Culture can be a killer. Our Africa regional coordinator in our office in Lilongwe, Malawi, reported on a "Church and Culture" conference he attended in 2005. Several city and country churches were represented at this event in Lilongwe. I was shocked to hear his report.

Among other unspeakable practices, I learned that it's quite common in rural communities to have a designated older man sexually initiate young women after their first menstrual period. Then each period thereafter requires another "specialist" who "cleanses" the girl through intercourse. If you have a handful of men "serving" several girls in a community, and if one or two or all of these men are HIV infected, well, you do the math. Even more troubling for me was hearing that the Church has no mitigating influence on these cultural practices. In fact, it tacitly endorses these sins against women by their silence. What's more, they have a few "cultural" practices of their own, like the provision of "Phoebes" for visiting preachers. The Apostle Paul in the book of Romans (16:1) refers to a personal assistant named Phoebe. Apparently Church culture in the countryside of Malawi has taken "personal assistant" to mean, "I prepare your food, I wash and mend your clothes, and if you wish, I sleep with you." To its credit, the conference roundly condemned all these practices and called the Church to account. "It's time to stop hiding behind culture," one speaker said. "Our 'culture' is destroying us."

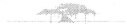

The Holy Grail for politically correct Western anthropologists, aid workers, and activists is "culture." "Don't mess with culture," they warn, a look of suspicion in their eye. They're especially nervous about "church" people intruding on the noble tradition and practices of ancient peoples. We're obviously blunt instruments with a triumphalist, spiritually colonizing agenda. We don't have the smarts or the sensitivity to blend in. We're simply looking for converts, regardless of any cultural "collateral damage."

Well, the fact is that HIV is messing with culture. Two of my staff had a most interesting meeting with an anthropologist in Nairobi in 2005.

"Have you seen this?" she asked, passing a two-page folder across the desk.

"What is it?" they asked.

"It's a Masai encyclical, for want of a better word," she smiled.

"See the pictures on the front and back? Each of those is the picture of a famous, revered Masai warrior. Their faces on the tract give it authority."

"What's it about?"

"It's a call to the Masai to change their centuries-old sexual culture. This, of course, is because of HIV/AIDS."

They were amazed at what it said. It decreed that Masai warriors were required to carry two condoms with them at all times, and to use them consistently whenever they had sex. They were not allowed to have penetrative sex with anyone but their wives. They were no longer required to offer their wives or daughters to visiting warriors. Boys, when going through their initiation ritual at age thirteen, were required to bring their own knives for their circumcision. Any noncompliance with these and many other new "rules" in the tract would culminate in punishments with varying degrees of severity. HIV/AIDS has radically changed the culture of one of the oldest tribes in Africa. Why? Because the Masai want to live.

"What about condoms?" I asked our meeting in Durban. "How effective are they?"

A doctor answered, "About as effective for HIV as they are for preventing pregnancy, about 85 percent to 95 percent effective."

"So you have a 5 to 10 percent chance of HIV infection if you use a condom?"

"That's about right with this caveat: you've got to use them every time, not just some of the time."

He went on to say that we Westerners, with our all-out promotion of condoms, had forgotten or neglected a few salient factors.

"First of all, you do a study with targeted groups of homosexuals in San Francisco on the effectiveness of condoms, and then project the findings to a general population on the other side of the ocean. Don't you see that general population dynamics are completely different from those of a specific, much smaller population of sexual lifestyles? Don't you understand that Africa is not America? That projecting from one culture to another, regardless of the good intentions, is an intrusion? Don't you see that most Africans see condoms as a foreign invention, something completely dissonant with their world?

"Why, some Africans see condoms as an American plot to reduce both their pleasure and their population! What's more, we can't afford condoms. And common sense will tell you that condoms must be used regularly, not irregularly. There has got to be buy-in on the part of the people, a consistent and constant supply, money to purchase them, and then consistent and constant use, otherwise condoms are a crock." "So why don't you tell us how you really feel," I thought.

At the time of this meeting, condoms were a sacred product—at least in terms of the West. And "experts" sneered at the Church with its wholesale rejection of safe sex via latex. A few years later even these skeptical experts had changed their tune. Now the buzzword is "safer sex." Even if the condom is effective 95 percent of the time with consistent use, what about the other 5 percent? Who wants to play Russian roulette with one's life?

The doctor was on a roll. Raising his voice with prophetic fervor, he lectured: "Really we're faced with two choices: risk avoidance or risk reduction. If you want to avoid HIV, you abstain from sex before marriage, and then you commit to faithfulness to your partner after marriage. In other words, no sex before or outside of marriage. Ever. If, on the other hand, you simply want to reduce risk, you use a condom. Consistent, and may I emphasize it again, consistent, use of condoms will certainly reduce risk, but it won't completely wipe it out. There's always that 5 percent lurking in the shadows."

He then went on to say that some of the preliminary study they were doing in Kwazulu Natal was suggesting that partner reduction was proving to be more effective than inconsistent condom use. "But bottom line," he asserted, "is behavior change." Apologizing for sounding like a preacher he said, "Kwazulu Natal and all of South Africa need a reintroduction to a biblical view of marriage." Then, looking at Kathy and me, he said, "That's why I think you're on the right track. But good luck. Most of the churches I know won't touch HIV/AIDS with a 10-foot pole."

An educator spoke next. "I agree," she said, "with the need for behavior change. But, before behavior can change, people need to know why they should change. I mean, we can see it, we know that pre- and extramarital sex is killing people. But many, many South Africans don't see it. They say, 'Why sex? We've been doing it for centuries. Why is sex the problem?' Many truly believe that America has poisoned them, or let loose some mad scientist's foul, avenging virus that will see us subjugated and dominated by the West. They need to be educated about HIV. We must get to the children twelve years of age and younger because twelve years is the average age of those becoming sexually active. They need to know what HIV is, how AIDS happens, how it can be avoided, and, in the process, perhaps most important of all, children need to be taught to accept personal sexual responsibility. If we succeed with this, we'll be well on our way to sustainable prevention."

After a pause, she continued: "We must not forget that most Africans are rural, religious, and traditional in their culture and world view. Even the educated city folk insist on being buried in their rural home community when they die. If we can build an educational platform that respects and reflects the essential goodness and God-fearing nature of Africa, I think we can go a long way in fighting this virus. With respect, we don't need or want an American solution. We want a 'made in Africa' solution. And," she said, looking at us, "that's why I think the local churches in Africa may be the key. They have more influence over children than any other entity in Africa today."

So there it was. Our job was cut out for us. We needed to be a Johnny Appleseed scattering seeds of HIV/AIDS awareness among the churches of southern Africa. Some seed, no doubt, would never germinate. Other seed would sprout quickly and die. Some would be stolen or defiled by political interference. But some would put down roots and thrive. I saw a day when Africa would be covered with "apple trees," local churches proactively engaged with the HIV/AIDS pandemic, providing sustainable shelter for orphans, widows, and all victims of the "avenging virus."

Thanks to the Durban consultation, we were now more than mere "do-gooders" breathing rarified air and sweeping into Africa with unimpeachable answers to their problems. We were now aware that there were multifaceted factors playing into any purported "solutions." Factors such as a migrating workforce, multiple sex partners, urbanization, poverty, the status of women, a silent Church, cultural practices, condoms, risk avoidance, risk reduction, education, and international dissonance. We realized that we were just at the beginning of a very steep learning curve. Two things mitigated our intimidation at the prospect: one, we had a sense of calling to this issue; and two, we weren't alone—everyone was a rookie when it came to HIV/AIDS.

As I sit here at my desk at home in Canada, writing these words, I look across the street to our neighbor's house. The woman who lives there is an invalid because of advanced multiple sclerosis. A young woman has just driven into the driveway and unloaded buckets, cleaning utensils, and a vacuum cleaner. She's going into the home to do the housework. She's a volunteer who comes faithfully every week. I silently bless her each time I see her. She's truly a servant and represents what is needed in the AIDS-inflicted areas of the world. Africa requires people with a servant's heart—people who aren't looking to aggrandize or find themselves. People who simply see that there's a job to do and do it for the sake of love. People who pick up the basin and the towel and humbly wash the feet of the suffering.

I've got to admit that this spirit of humble servanthood was a stretch for me. Sure, I had served the Lord and his people as a pastor and church planter. I had visited and prayed for the sick, comforted the grieving, rejoiced with the joyful, spent countless hours listening to the troubled, and all the other stuff associated with professional ministry. But I had never faced such a black hole as that presented by this horrific pandemic, a reality with a specific gravity that could suck the life out of you, obliterating your touch, your presence, your impact, your recognition by your peers for good work, a giant so huge and overwhelming that the only credit accruing to you for engaging it was survival. A tidal wave was not only threatening to swamp southern Africa, but it was also sure to drown all ego, hubris, arrogance, and self-confidence in billowing seas of destroyed lives. In other words, even though I was a reluctant servant, our voluntary entry into this horror forced us to lose ourselves for the sake of the lost. The only way to survive was by saving. The "pat-answer people" either perished in the first wave, or fled to the higher ground of conferences, seminars, and position papers. The irony was, and is, that the only way to live was to die.

And we've died a thousand deaths with more to come I'm sure. Let me give you a few examples.

Kathy and I are visiting a hospice in Johannesburg that cares for dying children. We enter the two-years-of-age-and-under ward. Kathy goes one way, I go the other. I look across the room and she is already holding an infant in her arms, cooing soft words, rocking from side to side. I turn to a crib in the corner.

A frail little girl sits there, looking up at me with large, empty eyes. A garish pair of red, heart-shaped sunglasses straddles her head. A feeding tube in one nostril is taped to her cheek. An intravenous drip is attached to her left arm and, dangling from each ear is a bright purple plastic earring.

"Hello, sweetheart," I say, bending down to look into her face. "Not feeling too well, huh?" I take her hand, and she slowly grips mine.

"Her name is Martha," a sister coming up behind me says (nurses in South Africa are "sisters"). Martha's grip tightens.

"Oh, what a lovely name." I turn to the sister, Martha now permanently latched to my hand.

"Yes, we named her. When she came here a year ago she had no name."

"Is she HIV positive?"

"Yes. Full-blown AIDS now. She has only a few weeks to live."

"How'd she get here?" I ask.

"A pastor brought her. Said he found her in a box beside her mother's grave."

"What!"

"Yes. He had finished performing another funeral, and discovered Martha on a fresh grave as he walked back to the cemetery entrance. He said he would have passed her by, but the box moved slightly as he glanced at it. He thinks some extended family member charged with the responsibility of caring for Martha decided to dump the baby, and abandoned her to die beside her mother. She was terribly dehydrated when she got here. We almost lost her the first day."

"But she rebounded?"

"Yes. Very well. For a time. But now her immune system is completely shot, and as I said, it's only a matter of time…" Her voice trailed away.

"Sister, before you go, does Martha have family or anyone who visits her?"

"No one. I'm sure she has relatives, but they don't know or don't care that they have her. She's a lost little soul and no one but us cares if she lives or dies."

I turn back to Martha. She still grips my hand. She looks at me, her eyes a little clearer now. I try to pray for her. I can't. There are no words, just a constricted throat and stinging tears. Her little hand is hot and dry. She is holding my finger tight, crying out to me: "Pick me up. Take me away. Hold me. Love me. I want to belong. I want to live."

I stand by her crib for several more minutes, holding her hand and unable to talk. We've connected, but I feel eclipsed by her suffering, staggered by her life experience, humbled by her dignity. I squeeze her hand, my grip saying, "Let me journey with you, let me carry you, you're so close, and I'm so far away." It took all my strength to gently, but firmly remove her hand from mine. I walked away, her heart gripping my heart, my thoughts dark, my soul sprained. If I could have died for her, I would have. I couldn't look back. Of all the thousands of suffering faces I have seen over these past few years in Africa, it is her face that stands out from the rest. And it's her grip that slays me still.

One day in Lilongwe, Malawi, we went to see the city cemetery. Our Africa regional coordinator took us there. On the way we drove down one street that was about half a mile long, and, within that distance we counted fourteen coffin-making establishments.

"Funerals are a growth industry," our host said. "Many pastors are burying two to three people a week."

I knew this was true. Just a few weeks previous an undertaker whom I happened to meet in a cemetery in East London, South Africa, told me that gravesites were becoming hard to find.

"We're trying to convince them to allow us to bury people vertically. It would make more space, and they would still be buried. But, they won't have it," he said, a touch of disgust in his voice.

"What about cremation?" I asked naively.

"Not a chance. No way. Would upset the ancestors."

We got to the old, central cemetery. To our shock and amazement, new graves had been dug between the graves of the past. On either side, and sometimes on the ends of the former graves lay new burial mounds covered with dry flowers and bric-a-brac from the departed's possessions. A gravedigger, working on another new one, stopped in his work to tell us that they had, in some cases, buried new caskets on top of old ones.

"Not exactly legal," he said, "but what can you do?"

As he resumed his work, we stood watching silently. All we could hear was his spade hitting the earth and the dirt being thrown up and out onto the old grave beside. Listening to this mournful sound I remembered the countless funeral processions we had seen throughout South Africa, Zambia, Zimbabwe, and Malawi. Somber groups of people, wearing their best clothes, singing hymns, walking slowly behind a casket to an open grave waiting in a field, or under a tree, and sometimes right beside the road. On occasion we had respectfully joined the mourners at the gravesite, in sympathy with the wailing and flailing, or struck dumb by the sight of the little children clustered around their mother's remains, feeling the pain, weeping not for loss but for sorrow, a little bit of ourselves dying. Then we walked past all the other new graves with their hand-painted memorials: "Alice, age 22, died November 3, 2002, in heavenly places"; "Jerome, 18 years, with God"; "Ezekiel, age 4, our angel." And on these mounds a plastic flower, an old dish rack, a toy bicycle, a wooden cross made out of sticks and wire. I'll never forget what rested on the grave of a little girl who had died at age four—a naked rubber doll with small twigs carefully attached to the head for hair. And, on its chest, a child, in crayon, had drawn a broken heart.

But it's not just the death and dying that kills you, it's the living death that you see everywhere—people living with relentless deprivation, food insecurity, grinding poverty, the burden of simply surviving driving them into the ground. How often have we seen little girls, six, seven, ten years of age with their infant siblings strapped to their backs? Sometimes they also have pails of water, or sticks of wood, or some other load balanced on their heads. The bone-thin, weary widows. The hovels they call home. The skin diseases. The distended bellies. The dust. The dirt. The sewage.

You can walk away from it—and you do because, unlike them, you can. But you can't forget. And you must come back. Again and again. You long for answers. Some way to stem the tide. You look across the heads of dusty children who have clustered around you and you see the humble little church building. There in the midst of the need is a candle flickering in the darkness. If we could fan that flame. If we could fuel it indefinitely. If the people who meet beneath its leaky roof could band together and let their light shine.

You see the church waiting to be reignited and hope suddenly stirs in your soul. Let God arise and let the Church rise with him.

Psalm 89 and Authentic Christianity

t's August 2003, twenty years after Kathy and I moved with our three children to Jerusalem. We had been invited by Israeli government officials in 1981 to establish a church in the Holy City (it was their idea, not ours!). Resigning from our church north of Toronto, we had moved to Jerusalem and spent the first year and a half developing a kibbutz volunteer program for North American students, and learning to speak Hebrew. We established the church in August 1983. So, here on the twentieth anniversary Sunday, Reverend Wayne Hilsden, my former associate, now senior pastor of King of Kings Assembly, has turned the pulpit over to me. Here is some of what I had to say:

> *The Hilsdens, Kathy, and I attended a* tish *at a Hassidic synagogue late Friday night. We arrived early, and walked the deserted streets of Mea Shearim for an hour or so. It seemed as though we had time-traveled back to eastern Europe in the nineteenth century and had entered a dark Polish ghetto. The streets, narrow, stone-paved, and dirty, were overshadowed by gray, featureless, small-windowed buildings housing shops and tiny residential flats. The windows above were lit, but cast no light on us below. They were open, however, and out of them cascaded the sounds of ultraorthodox families celebrating "Kabalat Shabat." The lilting resonance of the* Shabat *singing followed us with stereophonic effect as windows on either side of the narrow passageways sounded out their joy of the Lord's day. Then, we turned a corner where suddenly both street and windows were empty and soundless, with only a scrawny stray cat or an occasional shadowed, solitary, black-clothed figure quickly appearing and then disappearing in some darkened doorway.*

To say we felt a bit awkward would be an understatement. Our wives were dressed modestly and looked like modern, North American orthodox women. Wayne was wearing a dark suit and was looking passable, whereas I looked totally inappropriate in khaki slacks and shirt. The two of us, however, were dead giveaways in our brilliantly white kipot (skullcaps), which we'd picked up at the King David Hotel. Adding to our discomfort were the glaring signs stating, "Groups of tourists are highly offensive to our residents. You are not welcome to walk about our neighborhood viewing us as oddities. You must stop this practice now." Or, "Men and women in mixed company are not allowed beyond this gate."

So, with our wives following discreetly a few paces behind, Wayne and I, shielded by our pulsating kipot, forged ahead, hoping our feeble masquerade would not see us spray-painted by irate Shabat observers. We thought we were doing not too badly until we passed a street-level window where two five-year-old girls were sitting. They sweetly wished us "Shabat Shalom" and then asked us for money. Orthodox Jews never carry money on Shabat. These kids had instantly seen through our facade. They weren't fooled. So what would our welcome be like at the synagogue?

For Wayne and me, our arrival at the synagogue was a non-event. For Ann and Kathy, it was an incident. Orthodox women, of course, are not allowed to worship with the men. They are required to sit behind a curtain or shield either at the fringes of the main floor or up in a balcony. In this case, they entered at the back of the synagogue and climbed the stairs to a balcony where unaccountably some men were sitting. Ann and Kathy beat a hasty retreat, but the men were quicker. Shielding their eyes, the men pushed past our wives, and then Ann and Kathy returned to the balcony feeling conspicuous and leprous. Wayne and I, on the other hand, felt totally inconspicuous. In fact we felt invisible. The half-thousand or so black-coated men never once looked us in the eye. They looked around us and through us, but never at us. We might just as well have been ghosts.

About one hundred men were crammed into benches surrounding a long T-shaped table where the elders of the congregation sat. The benches spilled over onto sharply angled risers where another 400 men stood, awaiting the arrival of the rabbi. They were so tightly jammed together that there was no space between them at all. They looked like a uniform body of black gently bobbing back and forth in a supernatural breeze. And, as soon as the rabbi arrived, they broke out into a centuries-old minor-keyed chant that sounded otherworldly and stirred the soul.

We didn't stay for the whole service, but the general liturgy goes this way: They chant and sing for a half hour; the rabbi is given the wine and the bread along with a modest Shabat meal; he blesses the wine and then looks every man in the eye while saying "Le Chayim" (a very dramatic moment); each man then comes to the rabbi for a ceremonial bit of food; then they push back the benches and dance and sing until two or three o'clock in the morning. They've received their food from God and all is well.

What struck me as we stood among these Hasidim, invisibly as if we had come via a time machine, was how much and how little we have in common. And the essential distillation of "how much" and "how little" (setting cultural differences aside) is this: Like them we have a high view of the Word; unlike them we have a high view of the State of Israel. We are caught in the tension between the ancient and the modern. They live, in their radio and television-less world, as if the modern did not exist. And yet, as one modern, secular Israeli friend of mine put it, "They [the ultraorthodox] are 'the keepers of the flame.' They keep Judaism alive for the rest of us."

As a gentile I can't say whether my friend is right in his assertion. And in terms of the Word, which we, with the ultraorthodox, honor, I think we must acknowledge that the Talmud for them often takes precedence over the Torah, at least in terms of the quantity of time spent in study. But, as I stood there last Shabat, I was reminded of the root system from which my Christian faith springs, and the critical importance of the Old Testament. And my mind went back to the first seven years of this congregation's existence and my sermonic preoccupation with righteousness and justice—a preoccupation, by the way, which has influenced my life for the past thirty years.

Now, I know we all look at scripture through a "lens"—theologians call it a "hermeneutic," a way of interpreting. Interpretation can be, especially here in Jerusalem, very subjective and sometimes flaky. That's why we stress that you approach scripture with proven tools like a concordance, a Bible dictionary, and a trusted commentary or two—and that you always subject your interpretation to context, context, context. And, one must also allow the scripture to interpret itself. In order to do that, you must distill the essential truths of scripture for an interpretive foundation. My personal choice is Psalm 89 where the psalmist says, "Righteousness and justice are the foundation of thy throne, O God." This is the lens through which I read and interpret the Bible. As I see it, righteousness and justice are the essential DNA of who God is and what he expects of us.

I then went on to share with them the impact that our work in Africa was having upon us. We were seeing authentic Christianity rooted in concern for the broken, especially for the orphans and widows. A mere theological framework was now being "sheeted-in" with a superstructure of real faces, lives, and histories. Suddenly righteousness and justice were becoming an experience rather than a theory. We were on a steep learning curve, an adventure the likes of which we had never known before.

Chapter 3

Orphans and Widows:
Heaven's Chief Concern

*B*lessing is only seven years old. He looks five. With the entire school of 400 students behind him, he stands in front of us, squares his frail shoulders, and, in a voice loud and commanding enough to speak to hundreds, he says, "My name ees Blessing. I have a po-em for yoo."

> My motha' colled me Blessing
>   when I wass bawn.
> When I wass fo' she tol' me
>   I was a blessing from hayven.
> Then she died.
> My uncle he beet me evahree day
> Beet and beet
> I sleep outside at night
> One day he wass drunk and beet me
> Veddy bad
> He threw me in a deetch
> By the road
> Pasta Banda found me
> He picked me up
> He found a docta and heeled me
> Then he brought me to thees school
> I am veddy, veddy happy
>
> I am gong to be a pilot
> I thank God for Pasta
> He ees a fatha to me.

Kathy and I, and a few ministry colleagues, listened to this and many other "poems" that day at the Village of Hope at Racecourse just outside of Kitwe, Zambia. Time and again as the children told their stories, we were moved to tears. Beatings, rapes, poisonings(!), starvation, sickness, penetrating cold, loneliness, sadness, anger, bullying, dog attacks(!), and on and on, these children had faced these and other horrors. Just because they were orphans. Blessing's poem moved me the most—the last of his words struck like an arrow into my heart, "He ees a fatha to me."

Psalm 68:5 contains a pivotal, defining statement about God: "A father to the fatherless, a defender of widows, is God in his holy dwelling." The pastor who delivered Blessing from the ditch, stitched his wounds, and brought him to a "village" that houses, feeds, and schools him was truly "the father's hand extended," heaven reaching down. Blessing got it right: this pastor was a father to him. He was a representative of "the kingdom among" the poor and defenseless. The "village" was too. It was founded and funded by North American churches working with local Zambian churches. It is a model of righteousness and justice faithfully focused on the weakest link. More than a model, it's a home, a home for Blessing, his orphaned friends, and several widows serving as house mothers.

I've already stated in the introduction that HIV/AIDS is the greatest orphan- and widow-maker in history. It will continue to be so as the ratio of new infections and deaths rises. The millions of orphans and widows today will become hundreds of millions in this century. That's why Psalm 68:5 is so vital and relevant. It clearly states who God is—and he's never been more challenged to be who he is than today. We who call him "Father" have the awesome challenge to be father to these millions. So let's take our time and thoroughly examine this single sentence. Let's see what "father" and "fatherless" meant in Old Testament days. Let's do the same with "defender" and "widows." Let's get to the heart of this defining scripture so we can then, with knowledge, apply it to the greatest crisis in the story of mankind.

The Hebrew root for "father" is *ab* or *abh*. The word for "daddy" is *abba* (used in Israel to this day). It's most basic meaning is "a begetter." But it can also mean "ancestor, originator, chief." The first reference of *ab*, of course, is to one's immediate male ancestor, the person "out of whose loins" one has come. In Old Testament times, as progenitor or patriarch, he had inviolable status. He was honored and obeyed. His word was law.

The Father

An excellent biblical example of this comes from the story of Abraham and Isaac. It's a story about a father preparing to kill his son and burn his body as a sacrifice to God. It's as offensive a story as one can find in scripture. My only comfort comes from the knowledge that these were primitive times, and God dealt with the culture as it was, not with how it could have or should have been.

One of our sons, who pastors in Jerusalem, has a flat overlooking the Hinnom valley. Standing on his balcony, you look over the valley directly at Mount Zion. It's a million-dollar view. One day I was standing on that balcony, taking in the vista, when I suddenly found myself imagining what I would have seen a few thousand years ago.

First of all, I would have smelled something: the stench of garbage rotting and burning. The ancient Israelites used the Dung Gate on the south side of Jerusalem as a portal for dumping its waste into the valley. There it was consumed with constant "fire and brimstone," providing an everyday imagery for the netherworld, a Gehenna, where the lost suffered in the acrid heat of an oppressive hell.

Looking over to my left, to the southwest side of Jerusalem, I would have seen a huge altar-pyre, a "high place of Baal" (Jer. 32:35), called Topheth ("fireplace" in Aramaic), where the nation of Judah and the city of Jerusalem, first under King Ahaz, then King Manasseh, sacrificed and burned their firstborn children to the fire gods of Ammon and Moab. I imagined seeing a solemn procession of people, trumpets blaring, bells ringing, walking slowly but surely down to the evil pyre, a weeping mother and grim-faced father holding in his arms their first-born infant son, knowing that within minutes a priest would plunge a dagger into its little chest, and then with incantations and half-mad zeal, throw the lifeless but still warm corpse into the gaping jaws of the god Molech, to be consumed in the raging fires within its mouth. I saw the mother collapse with grief, and heard the father whisper into her ear, "We gave our firstborn for our transgressions, the fruit of our bodies for the sin of our souls" (Mic. 6:7b). I saw the other parents in the procession avert their eyes and turn to walk quickly away, shuddering at the horrific thought that it would only be a matter of time and it would be their turn. Others, who had already given their firstborn, lingered to comfort the distraught parents, their eyes blank and dark with memory.

These fire gods, Molech and Chemosh, traced their "lineage" back to the fire gods of the early Canaanites, whose culture and religious practices provided the social context in which we find Abraham in Genesis 22. Like the tragic couple at Topheth, the Canaanites had a great fear of the gods, and a profound conviction of their sins, so, they would sacrifice their beloved firstborn sons. They were reluctant but steady, crushed yet firm in their religious commitment and duty. It broke their hearts, but saved their souls.

If God says, "Take your son, your only son, Isaac, whom you love, and go to the region of Moriah. Sacrifice him there as a burnt offering on one of the mountains I will tell you about," (Gen. 22:2), how could Abraham do anything less? He had no way of knowing that God would surprise him with a substitute sacrifice, a ram, to take the place of Isaac. All he knew was that the God in whom he "believed" (Gen. 15:6) was awesome and was to be obeyed. As for Isaac, who was old enough to object and even to physically overcome his father, he knew that a father's authority was not to be questioned, even unto death.

In the Hebrew text the word for "boy" is n'r or na'ar, which means "boy, youth, servant." It has a wide range of application, from the infant Moses (Ex. 2:6) to the young adult Absolom (2 Sam. 14:21). Abraham refers to Isaac as a "boy" or "lad" (v. 5), but we need not think of "child" here. After all, Abraham was now well over 100 years old (anybody under 50 would be a "kid"!), and he had been living with Sarah and Isaac "in the land of the Philistines for a long time" (21:34). My guess is that Isaac was in his mid-20s. So why didn't he overpower his father when instructed to lay down on the altar Abraham had constructed? Why didn't he grab the knife as it was raised and run away? The only answer is that he believed his father's word had absolute authority. It would not have occurred to him to disobey. And maybe, just maybe, he had come to "believe" his father's God as well.

The point is this: In Old Testament times, a father had complete authority, total power. He could sell his children as slaves (Ex. 21:7). He could stone to death any of his family who tried to seduce him away from true faith to the worship of false gods (Deut. 13:6–10). And, any child who struck his father or mother, or who cursed them, was to be put to death (Ex. 21:15, 17). A father was a priest in his home (Gen. 17:23), both pastoring and protecting his children (Job 1:5). Mother and father were "the pride of their children" (Prov. 17:6b), and were to be honored (Ex. 20:12). Indeed, the fifth commandment to "honor" one's parents is "the first commandment with promise" (Eph. 6:2)—do this and you will "live long in the land." Parents were vital. Maybe this is why we have the seventh commandment, "You shall not commit adultery." The Almighty wants every child to be family-born.

"Father" may also refer to ancestors from years, even ages, past. Time and again we read about fathers (favorites are "my/your father Abraham" and "father David") who are several centuries removed from the times of those claiming descendant status. Sometimes "father" is an honorary term; other times it refers to the pioneer, the "founder" of societal categories such as "lyre and pipe" players, or "tent dwellers" (Gen. 4:20, 21).

Regardless of the application, "Father" is a powerful word. To have a father means to have a foundation, faithful support, protection, shelter, food, clothing, love, and a moral compass. It also means to have a home, a place where they always have to take you in. You have roots when you have a father. You know where you came from and you have a sense of identity. You belong.

This is what Blessing meant when he said his pastor/rescuer was a "fatha" to him. This father literally brought Blessing back from the grave. He filled Blessing's emptiness with every good thing. He not only gave him his life back, he gave him a life.

The Fatherless

God is a "father to the fatherless." He gives them a life. As his arm extended to a broken world, we who both fear and love him are to give a life to orphans. Not just a care package here, and a short-term missions team there (as important as they are), but a life. A life that can be lived for at least seventy years (when we get to the last chapter we'll discuss the "how"). A life with the dignity that having a father provides.

The word for "fatherless" in the Old Testament is *y-t-m* or *yatom*. Though the fatherless boy or girl may have had a mother, in Old Testament culture to be without a father was tragic. The fatherless had no economic anchor, no societal legitimacy, no hope of a future. So again and again the Old Testament prophets called on the people of Israel to step up and care for the fatherless. The fact that they failed at this consistently is underscored by the many excoriating prophetic words throughout scripture about this glaring social injustice.

Early on in scripture the Lord makes it clear that the fatherless (and their widowed mothers) have a very high place in his regard, and those who oppress them a very low place. "Do not take advantage of a widow or an orphan. If you do and they cry out to me, I will certainly hear their cry. My anger will be aroused, and I will kill you with the sword; your wives will become widows and your children fatherless" (Ex. 22:22–24).

A little later the author of Deuteronomy takes up the theme: "For the Lord your God is God of gods and Lord of lords, the great God, mighty and awesome, who shows no partiality and accepts no bribes. He defends the cause of the fatherless and the widow, and loves the alien, giving him food and clothing" (Deut. 10:17, 18). And, as in Exodus, there are strong words with regard to the treatment of "the alien, the fatherless, and the widow": "Do not deprive the alien or the fatherless of justice, or take the cloak of the widow as a pledge. Remember that you were slaves in Egypt and the Lord your God redeemed you from there. That is why I command you to do this. When you are harvesting in your field and you overlook a sheaf, do not go back to get it. Leave it for the alien, the fatherless and the widow, so that the Lord your God may bless you in all the work of your hands. When you beat the olives from your trees, do not go over the branches a second time. Leave what remains for the alien, the fatherless and the widow. When you harvest the grapes in your vineyard, do not go over the vines again. Leave what remains for the alien, the fatherless and the widow. Remember that you were slaves in Egypt. That is why I command you to do this" (Deut. 24:17–22). The Lord's stern words here are underscored by "you were slaves in Egypt." So, be sure you're empathetic and be warned: if you're not, you may become slaves in Egypt again.

The prophets and the psalmists are equally strong in their call for advocacy: "Stop doing wrong, learn to do right! Seek justice, encourage the oppressed. Defend the cause of the fatherless, plead the case of the widows" (Isa. 1:16b, 17). "If you really change your ways and your actions and deal with each other justly, if you do not oppress the alien, the fatherless or the widow and do not shed innocent blood in this place, and if you do not follow other gods to your own harm, then I will let you live in this place, in the land I gave your forefathers for ever and ever" (Jer. 7:5–7).

Zechariah had a sober word for God's people: "Administer true justice; show mercy and compassion to one another. Do not oppress the widow or the fatherless, the alien or the poor..." (Zech. 7:9). The consequence of not practising social justice is extreme: "'When I called, they did not listen; so when they called, I would not listen,' says the Lord Almighty. 'I scattered them with a whirlwind among the nations, where they were strangers. The land was left so desolate behind them that no one could come or go. This is how they made the pleasant land desolate'" (vv. 13–14). Because Israel wouldn't listen, because Israel was unjust, because Israel oppressed the weakest link, Israel was dispersed and the land became a wasteland. Harsh. Very harsh indeed. Israel forgot that everything God did for them, he did first and foremost "for his name's sake." Israel's neglect of social justice sullied God's name because his name—ha Shem—was inextricably linked to Israel. If Israel neglected the fatherless, God was neglecting the fatherless. And, bottom line, before God was anything in Israel, he was "the helper of the fatherless" (Ps. 10:14).

So, in God's eyes, the neglect and oppression of the fatherless was ground zero for injustice. Job, in bitter disappointment at his "comforters'" accusations, says of them, "You would even cast lots for the fatherless and barter away your friends" (Job 6:27).

The psalmist calls on God to "rise up, O Judge of the earth, pay back to the proud what they deserve." Why? Because "they slay the widow and the alien; they murder the fatherless" (Ps. 94:2, 6).

Isaiah vilifies Jerusalem:

> *See how the faithful city has become a harlot! She once was full of justice;*
> *righteousness used to dwell in her—but now murderers! Your silver has*
> *become dross, your choice wine is diluted with water. Your rulers are*
> *rebels, companions of thieves; they all love bribes and chase after gifts.*
> *They do not defend the cause of the fatherless; the widow's case does not*
> *come before them. (1:21–23)*

Seems that the erosion of righteousness and justice devalues a nation's view of human life, eviscerates the economy, and sets the stage for
drunkenness (you "dilute" the wine in order to drink more), rebellion,
thievery, corruption, and (the zenith of injustice) the total neglect of
the orphan and the widow. It appears that a nation's treatment of the
most easily preyed-upon is the litmus test for success or failure.

And, even though "fatherless" appears only once in the New Testament,
the words of James, the bishop of Jerusalem and Jesus's half-brother, keep
resonating: "Religion that God our Father accepts as pure and faultless
is this: to look after orphans and widows in their distress and to keep
oneself from being polluted by the world" (Jas. 1:27). You can't get away
from it in scripture: the priority of meeting the needs of the marginalized is the pivot point of true faith.

We've got to avoid the temptation of thinking that "true religion"
is something we fight for. Writing about it, arguing about it, even dying for it, can be empty and useless. The only thing that counts is living for it—perhaps more to the point, living it. Listen to the prophet
Malachi: "So I will come near to you for judgment. I will be quick to
testify against sorcerers, adulterers, and perjurers, against those who
defraud laborers or their wages, who oppress the widows and the fatherless, and deprive aliens of justice, but do not fear me, says the Lord
Almighty" (Mal. 3:5). Corrupt societies "mistreat the fatherless and
the widow" (Ezek. 22:7b) and "make widows their prey and rob the
fatherless" (Isa. 10:2b). Crumbling nations "drive away the orphan's
donkey and take the widow's ox in pledge" (Job 24:3). Like maraud-
ing vultures they pick the bones of the feeble. Self-consumption con-
sumes them, and expediency neutralizes moral values—"they make
friends with the terrors of darkness" (Job 24:17b). Justice stands in the

way of getting their way. So they turn a blind eye and willfully "thrust the needy from the path" (24:4). Against them the orphan and widow have no defense.

I don't know about you, but I need a break. This is pretty intense stuff. Time for a time-out. So, before carrying on with an exploration of Psalm 68:5, how about a brief discussion of the "great gulf fixed" between Old Testament culture and ours today? Perhaps I'll use the concept of "alien" as a case in point.

The Alien

As you may have noticed, Old Testament culture was patriarchal, raw, and primitive. When you read about fathers having the right to sell their daughters into slavery, you wonder if modern-day warlords in the Middle East aren't the rightful heirs to the Old Testament. And, regarding orphans and widows, we in the West have established a so-cial safety net to look after them. Our personal attention is not needed. We care for them at arm's length through our tax dollars.

This impersonal approach to social justice would never have been accepted in Old Testament times. A nation's strength was its social fab-ric, and the core fiber in that tapestry was the integrity of the extended family. The health of the family unit was the health of the nation. Father, mother, children, grandchildren, brothers, sisters, cousins, uncles, aunts, and their "accoutrements" were joined together in an unshakeable way. Their solidarity, family by family, built a great nation.

This is why the treatment of the orphan, widow, and alien was so critical. They were "outside" the camp. They didn't fit into the tight patriarchal family model. They were, in most cases, pathetic and po-tentially dangerous. Abject poverty combined with social rejection can create desperate people. Desperation can fuel social unrest and upheaval. The more prescient leaders could see gangs of orphans run-ning rampant, aliens robbing homes, raping, and murdering, widows begging in the streets, defenseless against sexual exploitation. The more compassionate saw these outsiders as an open wound in the body of the nation. They wanted to heal. There were, as well, those who saw these unfortunates as fodder for personal advantage. Steal the orphan's donkey, take liberties with the young widow, force the alien to work for nothing. And so, the alien, orphan, and widow were like a social mirror reflecting the true nature of individuals, families, and even the entire nation. Look at them and see yourself. Are you beautiful? Or are you ugly? The Old Testament culture, generally, said, "We want to be beautiful." Thus, they incorporated the alien, orphan, and widow into their family structure. We've been looking at the orphan and widow (and will continue to do so shortly), but let's look at the alien.

At the time of writing, Osama bin Laden, the world's most wanted man, is still at large. At the time of publishing I expect he'll still be in hiding. Why? Because he is probably under the protection of some Afghan warlord in a remote mountain hideout. In Afghani culture, any foreigner who puts himself under the protection of someone's "house" has a high, respectable status. And the master of that home will guard him to the death. He will protect him even if he is an enemy. Culture sets the protection of a guest as a core value, far above the more mundane responsibility of destroying an enemy.

The Hebrew word for "alien" in the Old Testament scriptures is *gr* (*ger*). Sometimes *yshv* (*yoshav, toshav*) is used. Both refer to a "sojourner, stranger, alien." A sojourner is a traveler who is between places and social categories. He's in a position of weakness because he's neither native-born nor a foreigner in the sense that he's ignorant of the culture in which he finds himself. But he lacks the protection and position of a native family. Therefore, until he is embraced by one, he's in a very vulnerable state.

The Old Testament culture recognized the fragility of the sojourner and did something about it. They took in the alien. They fed and watered him. They gave him clothing and a place to sleep. They did this not just to be nice, but because their culture taught that the sojourner had a legal claim to protection and full sustenance indefinitely. As for the fortunate stranger himself, he was expected to assume responsibilities and to add value to the household for as long as he was under its protection. Layabouts were frowned upon.

By the way, there was more than culture at work here. History played a huge role. Abraham, Lot, Isaac, Jacob, Esau, Joseph's brothers, David, and Elijah were all sojourners at one time or another in their lives. And, as the prophets make abundantly clear again and again, Israel was once a sojourner in Egypt. "Do not mistreat an alien or oppress him," warns Moses, "for you were aliens in Egypt" (Ex. 22:21). In the Ten Commandments, as listed in Deuteronomy (5:15), the Lord underscores his authority by reminding Israel "that you were slaves in Egypt and that the Lord your God brought you out of there with a mighty hand and an outstretched arm." What's more, Israel is not only required to do what is right for aliens, they are commanded to love them: "you are to love those who are aliens, for you yourselves were aliens in Egypt" (Deut. 10:19). And the God who delivered them is the protector of the vulnerable, especially the orphan, widow, and disinherited.

The Lord saw to it that the sojourner became a player in Israel's social fabric. Indeed, he was almost an Israelite: "Do not abhor an Edomite for he is your brother. Do not abhor an Egyptian, because you lived as an alien in his country. The third generation of children born to them may enter the assembly of the Lord" (Deut. 23:7, 8).

"Sojourner" in a profound way captured the very essence of Israel's relationship with God. They had been *hibaru* ("wanderers") until God had invited them into his "house" in his "land." They had entered into his protection and now, like all responsible sojourners, were trying to do the will of their (divine) host. When they forgot their status, the word of the Lord would ring down through the centuries: "The land must not be sold permanently, because the land is mine and you are but aliens and my tenants" (Ex. 25:23). True, you've lived there a long time, but remember, you're just leaseholders. To his credit, the one man who might have claimed ownership didn't. King David never forgot where he came from. "I dwell with you as an alien," he prayed, "a stranger, as all my fathers were" (Ps. 39:12b). So this is why the focus of social justice in Old Testament times always included the alien. Israel's history and culture demanded it.

Yes, there is a great gap between the culture of the Old Testament and our culture today. It would be impossible to attempt to replicate those ancient days. Even those who try fail (just ask the ultraorthodox Jews in Jerusalem how they're doing). *But the one enduring element that transcends time and bridges the huge chasm between now and then is the call to care for the alien, orphan, and widow.* Social justice is just as vital an issue today as it was yesterday. And, I believe, the Old Testament scriptures provide the very best way forward.

If we are going to care for the millions of orphans and widows that HIV/AIDS has created, we've got to master Psalm 68:5. Let's get back to it. We've discussed "father to the fatherless"; now, let's turn our attention to "defender of widows."

The Defender

Dayyan, from the Hebrew root *din* ("judge"), translated is "defender." It refers to someone who has the authority to administer justice by trying cases in law. Law is inferred. You can't administer justice without it. Israel, of course, had the Mosaic law at the very center of its being. History and culture may have described the ideal for life in Israel, but it took law to describe the meaning of life. It also took law to maintain that life. Law was the moral skeleton of Israel's vibrant existence.

As I've already pointed out, the meaning of life in Israel had everything to do with God's saving action in history. So the law was permeated with purpose: God intended to bless "all peoples on earth" (Gen. 12:3) through Israel. They were to be a nation with a world view and a world mandate. Law to bolster universal truth would be universally applied by a holy people, who would be "a light [to] the Gentiles" (Isa. 49:6). They were to be "blameless before the Lord your God" (Deut. 18:13). In this sense Israel was being shaped by law to be a priest to the world, a mediating influence between heaven and earth. To this end the law also maintained life in Israel by legislating holiness and punishing unholy behavior. This is why there are 613 laws—the Ten Commandments at the core—but everything else a nomadic people needed to maintain physical and spiritual holiness through years of desert wanderings. Needless to say, the complexity of understanding and applying these hundreds of laws required experience, wisdom, age, and authority. This is where the "judge" or "defender" came in.

The book of Deuteronomy, more than any other Old Testament book, establishes the DNA of Israel's life in the world. Moses instructs the people in great detail about everything from sex to prayer, including what is expected of judges. He says, "Appoint judges and officials for each of your tribes in every town the Lord your God is giving you, and they shall judge the people fairly. Do not pervert justice or show partiality. Do not accept a bribe, for a bribe blinds the eyes of the wise and twists the words of the righteous. Follow justice and justice alone, so that you may live and possess the land the Lord your God is giving you" (Deut. 16:18–20). The judge was to execute absolute justice, which meant impartiality and a resistance to making popular judgments. And, unlike some witnesses in lawsuits, he was to beware the influence of the crowd, and even the manipulative skills of the downtrodden. "When you give testimony in a lawsuit, do not pervert justice by siding with the crowd, and do not show favoritism to a poor man in his lawsuit" (Ex. 23:2, 3). The image of the blindfolded judge holding the scales of justice comes to mind. He was to be objectivity and justice personified.

The ultimate judge, of course, is none other than God himself. First of all, he is judge over all the earth: "Rise up, O Judge of the earth; pay back to the proud what they deserve" (Ps. 94:2). He is also judge of the nations: "He will judge between the nations and will settle disputes for many peoples. They will beat their swords into plowshares and their spears into pruning hooks. Nation will not take up sword against nation, nor will they train for war anymore" (Isa. 2:4). Then he judges his chosen ones: "He summons the heavens above, and the earth, that he may judge his people: 'Gather to me my consecrated ones, who made a covenant with me by sacrifice.' And the heavens proclaim his righteousness, for God himself is judge" (Ps. 50:4–6). And, as King David himself prayed, God is judge of the individual: "Arise, O lord, in your anger; rise up against the rage of my enemies. Awake, my God; decree justice. Let the assembled peoples gather around you. Rule over them from on high; let the Lord judge the peoples. Judge me, O Lord, according to my righteousness, according to my integrity, O Most High. O righteous God, who searches minds and hearts, bring to an end the violence of the wicked and make the righteous secure" (Ps. 7:6–9). And it is this judge who declares himself defender of the weak.

The point of the defender's advocacy for the widow was more than achieving temporal justice for her. It saw beyond redress to the rest of her life. The judge, as interpreter of the law, knew that the ultimate purpose was a long, fruitful fellowship with God. The law was not to be seen as a legalistic system, but as the genetic code for abundant life. Defending widows meant providing them with both short-term and long-term hope. Justice for her meant she would sleep well at night.

The Ten Words

The Law, or "Torah" as it is called to this day (from *y-r-h* or *yarah*— "throw, cast, shout, teach") is found in the first five books of the Bible (the Mosaic Law or Law of Moses), and provides the infrastructure for proper judgments. At its very core is what we popularly know as the Ten Commandments. To understand the work of a defender in Israel, we've got to understand these commandments. Let's take a look.

20 *And God spoke all these words:*

> ²*"I am the Lord your God, who brought you out of Egypt, out of the land of slavery.*
> ³*You shall have no other gods before me.*
> ⁴*You shall not make for yourself an idol in the form of anything in heaven above or on the earth beneath or in the waters below.* ⁵*You shall not bow down to them or worship them; for I, the Lord your God, am a jealous God, punishing the children for the sin of the fathers to the third and fourth generation of those who hate me,* ⁶*but showing love to a thousand generations of those who love me and keep my commandments.*
>
> ⁷*You shall not misuse the name of the Lord your God, for the Lord will not hold anyone guiltless who misuses his name.*

*[8]Remember the Sabbath day by keeping it
holy. [9]Six days you shall labor
and do all your work, [10]but the
seventh day is a Sabbath to the
Lord your God. On it you shall
not do any work, neither you,
nor your son or daughter, nor your
manservant or maidservant,
nor your animals, nor the alien
within your gates. [11]For in six
days the Lord made the heavens
and the earth, the sea, and all
that is in them, but he rested
on the seventh day. Therefore the
Lord blessed the Sabbath day
and made it holy.
[12]Honor your father and your mother, so that
you may live long in the land
the Lord your God is giving you.
[13]"You shall not murder.
[14]"You shall not commit adultery.
[15]"You shall not steal.
[16]"You shall not give false testimony against
your neighbor.
[17]"You shall not covet your neighbor's house.
You shall not covet your
neighbor's wife, or his manservant
or maidservant, his ox or
donkey, or anything that belongs to
your neighbor." (Ex. 20:1–17)*

These words, coming as they did after several weeks of lightning, thunder, smoke, and mystery on Mount Sinai, found the people so intimidated that they said to Moses: "Speak to us yourself and we will listen. But do not have God speak to us or we will die" (Ex. 20:19). They understood that their lives would never be the same if they lived.

So, what scared them? Before I answer, let me tell you about my personal experience with fright and delight on Mount Sinai.

It was two in the morning when we got the wake-up call. My camera crew and I had traveled the day previous from Eilat in southern Israel to the foot of Mount Sinai. We had spent several lively hours negotiating with the village headman about the cost and number of camels we would need to transport us and our equipment up the mountain in the early hours of the next morning. That morning had come. Bleary-eyed but excited, we stumbled out of our modest hostel into the darkness and said hello to nine cud-chewing, homely, and slightly "off" camels. Their handlers, wearing *kaffiyehs* and robes, squatted in a huddle around an open fire, brewing nasty-looking pitch they called coffee. They kindly offered us small cups of the stuff, and I was the only one of our team who accepted. I did say no, however, to the offer of a foul-smelling Gitanes cigarette. We were keen to get on with the three-and-a-half-hour trek to the top of Mount Sinai. We wanted to be at the summit for the most stunning sunrise in the world. Then, with the breathtaking backdrop of the Sinai range, we would spend the day taping segments for a national television show. But first we had to get on those camels.

Before you can sit on a camel, you've got to get the camel to sit on the ground. Sounds easy, but it isn't. The handler makes a soft clucking noise in his throat, the camel responds with a fingernails-on-the-blackboard bray of protest, baring his teeth, expressing contempt for the idea with a significant volume of spittle. The handler quietly insists. The camel persists. The handler reveals the whip from the folds of his robe. The camel blinks his heavily lidded eyes in reluctant acceptance of his fate, grunts loudly, and plops himself awkwardly on his knees, his hump and rump still high in the air. Then, disjointed like a trailer behind a tractor, the back end follows suit, hitting the ground with a small cloud of dust and nether flatus. Braying again and grinding his long yellow teeth in defeat, the camel glares at his master, then turns his long-eyelashed malevolence on you. He's daring you to even think, let alone try, to climb onto his back.

Honor demands you do it, rather than yield to a cowardly comment like, "Ya know what? I think it's a lovely morning for a walk!" The hump, with its strange two-horned saddle atop what can only be described as a turkish carpet, awaits. You grab the first horn and swing your leg over the other horn, careful to avoid embarrassment and injury, and voila! You're on. The handler instructs you to hook one leg around the front horn and lock it with the other leg by crossing your ankles. Meanwhile, the owner of the gelatinous mass on which you are precariously perched is turning his head from side to side, looking to bite you.

The handler gives a guttural cluck, the camel responds with another burst of braying, grunting, teeth gnashing, and spitting (all of which you can now feel through the saddle), and suddenly, without warning, his back end rises to its full height, hurtling you forward with enough force to throw you head over heels to the ground. Even as you grab the front horn in panic, his front end rises with equal force, throwing you backward, the rear horn impaling your lower back. Your life flashes before your eyes. When you open them, you're sitting like a king on a mountain, master of all you survey. Your thoughts, however, are anything but regal; you wonder darkly when it will be, over the next few hours, that the camel will get its revenge.

Soon everyone is seated atop hostile hills of dromedary. Several camels are loaded with television equipment strapped to the horns of their riderless saddles. The lead handler gives a cluck and nine camels lumber off into the night. Like ghostly galleons in shimmering starlight, our caravan stretches out on the plain, Mount Sinai a silent, brooding darkness on the far horizon.

When you're sitting in a small boat, the wave action of the water raises and lowers it in a regular but gentle fashion. It's very similar to riding a camel. But in this case the motion of the camel rocks you gently forward and backward, forward and backward, forward and backward, the only sound the muffled planting of large desert-adapted camel feet on the sand. When you're sleep-deprived, as we were, it's enough to rock you to sleep.

It took about forty minutes to cross the plain to the foot of Mount Sinai. As we approached the darkened walls of the Santa Katarina monastery, I looked around at the desert expanse we had just traversed in the moonlight and saw that it was like an island of flat, featureless sand in the midst of hulking quartz sentinels. It was only about 3 miles by 5 miles in size, and I could imagine it covered with the tents and campfires of the children of Israel. It was here they waited for the man of God to come down from the angry, fulminating mountain. It was here the words would be spoken that would change the world.

Passing the silent monastery, we began a gentle climb. For about an hour it was fairly straightforward—nothing but the four-footed plodding of our now quiescent beasts and the occasional clucking of the handlers. Each of us was lost in his own thoughts. There were no comments, no words exchanged, just a velvet, magical carpet ride.

I hardly noticed the first switchback. Or the next. I was so lost in the massive size and nearness of the brilliant Sinai stars (no light pollution), the surreal rhythm of the riding motion, the air, the walls of stone, and the romance of the moment, that I failed to notice we had suddenly attained a great height. As we reached the third switchback, I happened to look down. This was a mistake.

I was looking at a 1,500-foot drop. On my right I could reach out and touch the mountain, on my left a fall to certain death. And there was my camel's left front foot about 6 inches from the edge. My heart was in my mouth. I felt caught between time and eternity. I remembered the evil gleam in the camel's eye a few hours ago and wondered if payback time was now. But it wasn't. As if he was on autopilot, the camel sure-footed it for another terrifying hour up, up, and up. He didn't miss a beat, even while my heart missed several. Two-thirds of the way up we stopped. The camels could go no farther. From here we'd have to shoulder the equipment and climb the remaining 2,000 feet under our own power. It was a daunting and exhausting ascent.

After an hour of lungs burning, legs like jelly, three steps and rest, three steps and rest, three steps and rest, we made the summit. The dark sky was beginning to give way to a thin light in the east as we flung our equipment and ourselves to the ground, gasping for breath in the almost empty air. As we regained our strength, the sky continued to lighten.

At a word from our guide we stood. We could now see the entire Sinai range. From horizon to horizon the jagged mountains thrust their ancient heads into the heavens. Even as we watched in wonder they began to change color. In a matter of a few minutes they all were transformed from a dirty brown/black to a burnt three-dimensional red. Then they became brilliant pink. The wonder of the sight was so awesome I found it hard to breathe. There were no words. We just stood there and stared. It took about ten minutes for the sun to break above the horizon. As it did the color began to fade. With it we began to breathe again. Then came the words. The exclamations. The looks at one another. Together we had shared one of the most magnificent sights in the world.

Moses saw many of those sunrises: "The Lord descended to the top of Mount Sinai and called Moses to the top of the mountain. So Moses went up..." (Ex. 19:20). And more magnificent than any of them was the overwhelming presence of God himself, who "descended" to the summit. On one of those descents God had said to the ascender, "You yourselves have seen what I did to Egypt, and how I carried you on eagles' wings and brought you to myself. Now if you obey me fully and keep my covenant, then out of all nations you will be my treasured possession. Although the whole earth is mine, you will be for me a kingdom of priests and a holy nation" (vv. 4–6). Here on the top of Sinai, God gave Moses the ten words that would provide the DNA for a priestly nation, the path that would forever describe the ascent to holiness from unholiness, the genetic code that would ultimately shape Isaiah's vision that "a shoot will come up from the stump of Jesse; from his roots a Branch will bear fruit" (Isa. 11:1). Israel's messiah, who would one day "judge the needy with righteousness" and "give decisions for the poor with justice" (v. 4), would trace the roots of his ministry to a sunrise over Sinai.

The people, however, saw no morning light: "Mount Sinai was covered with smoke, because the Lord descended on it in fire. The smoke billowed up from it like smoke from a furnace, the whole mountain trembled violently, and the sound of the trumpet grew louder and louder" (Isa. 18–19). What they saw and felt was terrifying. It seemed they were about to be engulfed in a volcanic eruption. It's a wonder they didn't flee in fear.

Then came the ten words—action words—for the Law is God in action. First things first: "I am the Lord your God, who brought you out of Egypt. ..." Don't forget me, says the Lord. You know me. I'm the God of the exodus. The pivot point of your history is there. What you're about to hear will make you holy. You must "be holy, because I am holy" (Lev. 11:45). So don't forget. Here's the deal:

> No other gods
> No idols
> No misuse of my name
> Remember to keep the Sabbath holy
> Honor your parents
> No murder
> No adultery
> No stealing
> No false testimony about your neighbor
> No coveting anything of your neighbor's

Or, more succinctly yet:

> *no gods, no idols, no blasphemy, holy Sabbaths, honored parents, no murder, no adultery, no stealing, no lying, no coveting*

And in ten words:

> *gods, idols, blasphemy, Sabbath, parents, murder, adultery, stealing, lying, coveting*

Remember these words, and the other words these ten bring to mind, and you'll be on your way to becoming the nation of priests I want you to be. The table is set.

The defenders of the weak worked from this ten-word grid. They eschewed a low view of family (adultery, coveting), a low view of property (stealing), a low view of life (murder), a low view of truth (lying), a lack of gratitude (coveting), and judged on the basis of a high view of neighbor that abrogated injustice and provided their defendants with personal worth and dignity. They prioritized a view of history that valued those who had gone before (parents), especially the one who had delivered them from Egypt. Their deliverer's name described his unique unity and must not be misused for magic, by rote, thoughtlessly, or as a means to an end (gods, idols, blasphemy). They protected the weekly day of memory and rest (Sabbath). As they weighed the balances with these ten weights, the orphan and widow found themselves protected, defended, and energized with hope. When, for whatever reason, these vulnerable ones were left defenseless, Elohe Yisrael himself took the seat of judgment. Justice was to rule both strong and weak, honored and dishonored, rich and poor. No one was to be left behind. This was the genius, the righteousness, the justice of the ten words.

The Genius of Tithing

These words seeded whole sentences, paragraphs, and books as time went on. Some of those emerging laws dealt specifically with the defense of widows. But generally she was included in the trilogy of "orphans, widows, and aliens." Here's one of those laws. It's about tithing and prevailed for centuries: "At the end of every three years, bring all the tithes of that year's produce and store it in your towns, so that the Levites (who have no allotment or inheritance of their own) and the aliens, the fatherless, and the widows who live in your towns may come and eat and be satisfied, and so that the Lord your God may bless you in all the work of your hands" (Deut. 14:28, 29). Later in the same book we read, "When you have finished setting aside a tenth of all your produce in the third year, the year of the tithe, you shall give it to the Levite, the alien, the fatherless, and the widow. … Then say to the Lord your God: 'I have removed from my house the sacred portion and have given it to the Levite, the alien, the fatherless, and the widow, according to all you commanded. I have not turned aside from your commands nor have I forgotten any of them'" (26:12, 13).

Tithing simply referred to "a tenth." Every year the Israelites were required to bring a tenth of their produce and flocks to Jerusalem (Deut. 12:5, 17). The tithe was seen as "holy to the Lord." So, the Israelite was commanded to bring "a tithe of everything from the land, whether grain from the soil or fruit from the trees [which] belongs to the Lord; it is holy to the Lord. If a man redeems any of his tithe, he must add a fifth of the value to it. The entire tithe of the herd and flock—every tenth animal that passes under the shepherd's rod—will be holy to the Lord" (Lev. 27:30–32).

When the tithe got to Jerusalem it was to be given to the temple workers, the Levites. Because they were involved in sacred work, the Levites had no income from conventional means, and were to be supported with "the tithes that the Israelites present as an offering to the Lord" (Num. 18:24). Then the Levites were to give a tenth of the tenth as a sacrifice to the Lord, and sustain themselves with the rest. Every third year, "the year of the tithe," the Israelites were to stockpile their tithes in their own towns and villages, where a sort of depot was situated in order to meet the needs of "orphans, widows, and aliens." Thus the reference to Deuteronomy 14 a few paragraphs back. (Josephus, the Jewish historian, refers to this tithe as "the poor tithe," and says it became a yearly tithe.) Suffice it to say that this law of the tithe provided a significant social safety net for the poor. It was an extension of "the ten words" that had profound social justice implications.

So, through "his words in action," the Lord became a "father to the fatherless" and "a defender of widows." The Achilles' heel of this provision, of course, was the attention or neglect of his people in terms of obeying his "commands" regarding the collection and equitable distribution of the tithe. Sometimes, in extreme situations, the Lord would directly intervene (see the story of the widow of Zarephath in 1 Kings 17:7–24). But his law required that Israel, unlike corrupt societies who "mistreat the fatherless and the widow" (Ezek. 22:7b), and "make widows their prey and rob the fatherless" (Isa. 10:2b), be sure to watch "over the alien and sustain(s) the fatherless and the widow" (Ps. 146: 9). God, by his words and his actions, directly or by extension through his people, was committed to providing daily necessities for the vulnerable and executing "justice on their behalf" (Deut. 10:18). They were a part of the whole, and the Most High in his holiness was holistic in his care.

The Soiled Ragdoll

Late one evening in South Africa, Kathy and I did something we had determined, through experience, never to do again. We drove at night. We had had so many dramas, lip-biting moments, and near misses on Africa's roads at night that we had become daytime travelers exclusively. It was just too scary navigating unlit, narrow roads, littered with jarring potholes, some deep enough to be filled with water and children playing in them. No kidding. See for yourself the next time you're driving the roads around Maputo, Mozambique. They were criss-crossed by endless streams of goats, dogs, and people, shoulderless, plagued with out-of-camber curves, and whatever else you can think of that threatens life and limb. Try stalled trucks (or lorries as they're called). They have no warning lights or reflectors. They simply leave the truck in the way, with a thin, leafy branch torn from a tree placed on the road about thirty feet in front and back. In the black of night you're expected to see and avoid this wall of steel and rubber. Then, God forbid, if you should hit a pedestrian, you're told to keep driving to the nearest police station (who knows where it is?), report the accident, and drive hurriedly away (lest the gathered mob kill you—an "instant justice" reflex).

Kathy and I saw this happen one night in Zimbabwe. We'll never forget the resigned horror on the face of the driver as a group of about twenty angry young men roughly hauled him away from a petrol station to which he had fled. He knew he was going to die. And, if you should come on an accident with bodies lying on the road, you're counseled to stay away. It could be a setup. You stop and thieves emerge from hiding. You're beaten and robbed. Or, if there is blood, it's probably HIV-tainted, so don't touch it. It's better to pass by on the other side. Or so the Africans tell us.

This particular night we were driving to our hotel from a major pastors' conference where I had been speaking about the Church and its responsibility to care for HIV/AIDS orphans and widows. We had stopped at a stop sign in the village adjacent to the conference center. As I was about to accelerate through the intersection, Kathy grabbed my arm.

"Isn't that a body?" she exclaimed.

"Where?"

"Over there." She pointed across the intersection.

Sure enough, there was a small body lying on the road in a fetal position right up against the curb. It was surrounded with what looked like a pool of blood. My gut wrenched. What should we do? Heed the warnings? Mob. Thieves. HIV. Find the police station? Where? Pass by and forget it? These thoughts flashed by in a millisecond. Then I remembered the restaurant.

Just 200 yards past the body was a restaurant where Kathy and I had eaten lunch that day; maybe it was still open. They had a phone and could call the police. I sped off. Slamming on the brakes in the parking lot I rushed into the dining room, ran to the bar, and in moments the bartender was calling the police. I returned to the car and tore off back to the body. I wasn't thinking now. The visceral had overtaken the rational. My gut instinct was in charge.

I stopped mere feet away from the inert form, the headlights casting everything in stark relief. As I got out of the car Kathy said, "Be careful." Walking up to the body the first thing I noticed was that the pool of blood wasn't blood. It was some other bodily fluid, probably urine. Then I saw that this person, small though she was, was not a child but a woman. I smelled alcohol.

I bent down and touched her face. She groaned. She was alive! Gently I picked her up, soiled and ragdollish, and propped her beside me against the fence. Then I asked a stupid question.

"Are you okay?"

No answer. Then, another foolish act, I reached into my pocket to find some money for her. Obviously I was under the influence of adrenaline. She half-opened her eyes.

I looked for cuts, bruises, broken bones. Again I asked, "Are you okay?"

"Ya-yes, baas. I be okay," she mumbled.

Drunk. She's drunk. She'd not been hit by a car. She'd just passed out. Relief. There's the broken whiskey bottle over there.

"Can I pray with you?" I asked.

"Yes, please."

I prayed. She looked at me, more clearly now, and said, "You a good man. Man of God."

Just then, to my amazement, the police arrived. The senior officer rushed up to us, looked past me, and said, "Oh! Lulu, how are we tonight?"

"You know her?" I asked.

"Very well," he answered. "She's a widow who lives a few kilometers from here. Got four kids. She works three jobs. A good woman. Drinks too much, but who can blame her for wanting to escape the pain from time to time?"

"Will you take her home?" I asked.

"Sure will. We'll take good care of her."

I picked her up. She felt like a child. I took her to the police van. As I did I noticed several pastors from the conference had stopped and were watching us with large eyes. I nodded at them. The police drove off and I returned to our car.

After a quick summary of everything to Kathy, she said, "Did you see those pastors?"

"I did. They looked a bit shocked."

"What? To see a white guy stopping to help someone lying on the road?"

"Maybe."

"Maybe they were surprised to see you practising what you preached tonight."

Oh yeah. I had preached about the Church walking by on the other side as HIV/AIDS victims lie dying. The parable of the Good Samaritan relevant to the age.

"Good thing you stopped, huh?"

"Yeah."

As we drove away I noticed that my shirt was wet, and I smelled of urine and whiskey. I can smell it to this day.

Hosea encourages Israel to return to the Lord with this prayer:

Forgive all our sins
and receive us graciously,
> *that we may offer the fruit of our*
> > *lips.*
Assyria cannot save us;
> *we will not mount war-horses.*
We will never again say, 'our gods'
> *to what our own hands have*
> > *made,*
> *for in you the fatherless find*
> > *compassion. (14:2b, 3)*

"Sound the Alarm, Donya."

*P*eople often ask me where I'm from. With tongue in cheek I answer, "Airplanes." It seems our life is a blur of airports, passport control, and customs desks, with several airport tax or departure tax kiosks in the mix—"That will be $35, sir." (US dollars, of course.)

Kathy and I have flown in all kinds of planes from every size, shape, and color of airport. We've flown twenty-two-hour flights and two-hour flights, daytime and nighttime, and sometimes the condition of the airplanes (third- and fourth-hand with some African airlines) has given us pause. I remember one plane in Tanzania where the seat backs were held in place with duct tape (color-coded, mind you). The fiberglass frames of the seats were full of stress cracks. "I wonder how many stress fractures there are in the wings," I thought. Then there are the landings. One two-attempt landing during a mini-hurricane in Dakar comes to mind, but I'll never forget the one in Tegucigalpa, Honduras.

I was flying into this Central American country at the request of the First Lady. She had become aware of the encroaching threat of widespread HIV in her nation, and was determined to do something about it. She had heard about our vision, "Every Church a Mother Teresa," and felt that her very religious people needed to be engaged in fighting HIV church by church. She also wanted to hear about what we'd learned in Africa. So, there I was, flying from Toronto via Miami, about to experience a landing unlike any I'd had before.

Usually a landing strip can be seen from far away, and a gentle, gradual descent takes place over the course of an uneventful 120 miles or so.

Airport locations are chosen for this purpose. Mountains, hills, or any other vertical obstacle present obvious dangers, especially in poor visibility or bad weather. This is why you don't see airports built in mountainous regions.

But what do you do when an entire country is mountainous? What do you do when the capital city is built on the sides of those mountains and the only level spots are the bottom of steep-sided valleys? You choose the lesser of several bad options and build an airport, hoping that the pilots will have the skills to touch down in a very difficult location. And air traffic controllers, flight crews, and passengers who have been this way before pray a lot.

I, of course, was a naif. Calmly reading a book, I was oblivious until the first sudden drop in combination with a steep bank left caught my attention. I looked out and to my astonishment it appeared we were almost bouncing off a mountaintop. Then another quick turn, another mountaintop, another bank, another mountain. "Are we about to crash?" I thought, my grip tightening on the armrests. A quick dip, we're skimming rooftops, then a highway appears right beside us. "We're landing on a road!" Then touchdown, cars streaming along beside us. "We're okay," I think. Yes. We're okay. We've landed—at the airport. On the way off the plane the crew members are clustered near the door to the cockpit. I say to the pilot, "Dicey landing."

"Yep, sure is. Every time. When you land in Tegucigalpa you've got to fly the plane." I walked to passport control in gratitude and silence. Gratitude for a pilot who had somehow succeeded; silence at the vulnerability we all share. My heart stopped pounding after customs.

The leader of an international women's organization and her driver meet me at the gate. She has facilitated this meeting with the First Lady and has news. She tells me the meeting has moved from Tegucigalpa to San Pedro Sula.

"How far is that?" I ask.

"Oh, about a five-hour drive."

Great. I've been traveling by air for six hours, now by car for another five or so. Well, at least I'll get to see some of the country.

And what a country! Up, down, up, around, down, up, up again, pass the exhaust-belching truck, near miss, "Didn't see that car through the smoke," explains the driver, down, down, around, a long line of trucks, pass, near miss again, different explanation, dramatic, breathtaking scenery, up, up. I smiled wryly, remembering the landing at Tegucigalpa, which was child's play compared to this driving. But at least I'd experienced bad roads, bad traffic, and bad driving many times in Africa. The only difference was that here in Honduras there weren't endless streams of people walking on the shoulders of the roads. The Hondurans appeared to be a bit better off. I ask about this and the driver says, "Annual income per worker is about $1,000 US a year." Three times that of the average African. And it shows. There's poverty everywhere, but it looks better here than in Africa.

We arrive in San Pedro Sula in the late afternoon. We check in at the hotel, and I'm told the First Lady will meet us in a small conference room at 7:30. Time for a shower and a nap. I can't nap. I'm wired, as my kids say—the flight, the landing, the drive, the conversation, the novelty, the excitement, the nervousness at meeting the president's wife, all these combine to make sleep impossible. But I have time to shower and to think.

"This is a new one," I say to myself. "We've always worked from the ground up with churches. Here it looks like we're engaging from the top down. Sure, lots of leaders, government officials, even a prime minister or two have shown interest in our work, but this is the first time we've seen a First Family want to take initiative. But we work with churches—that's our specialty. How can I engage the state with the church here? Strange bedfellows. But that's what AIDS is doing. It's forcing people out of the box. The conventional barriers, borders, and protocols are stressing and fracturing under the weight of the death culture precipitated by the pandemic. Don't forget to mention to her your vision of the Church as the delivery mechanism for HIV/AIDS proactivity. Show her that the Church may be her greatest ally in the fight ahead. What do I call her? Your Ladyship? Your Excellency? Ma'am? Maybe she'll tell me."

"Call me Donya," she says as she sweeps into the room. Strong, athletically built, and beautiful, she looks at me with large, deep brown eyes. "Welcome, Pastor. I've looked forward to meeting you." Her personal secretary and her sister are with her. Her sister is a physician. We get right to it.

She begins by telling us that she has just returned from New York where she met with the secretary general of the United Nations. She told him of her grave concern about HIV/AIDS in Honduras and that she could not stand aside and let it continue to kill her people. She didn't know what she was going to do, but she was going to do something. Her dark eyes flashing, she says, "He told me he and the UN would help me. 'Decide what you're going to do and we'll back you.' he said. So we must do something right away. This is why I wanted to talk to you, Pastor, and I apologize for the suddenness of the invitation and appreciate that you made the effort to get here quickly."

"What is the prevalence of HIV/AIDS in Honduras?" I ask.

"The official statistics have it at 2 percent," she answers, "but we know it's much, much worse. The point is we don't want it to get as bad as those African nations. We want to nip it in the bud."

I agree that the statistical evidence doesn't give an accurate picture anywhere. Almost all the stats are based on prenatal tests of pregnant women. There is very little reliable study of men, women who aren't pregnant, teens, and children. Thus, any stats must be taken as very conservative at best, and inaccurate at worst.

"Why do you believe it's much worse?" I ask.

"Because of the thousands of rural and poor people who are sick," she says. "We're beginning to see a dark cloud arising. Please, Pastor, tell us about Africa."

So I began. I gave her a quick overview of the latest UN statistics about the exponential growth of HIV/AIDS in southern Africa over the past decade. I talked about declining life expectancy, the daily new infections with HIV, the daily numbers of young people dying, the disproportionate numbers of young women and girls infected, the millions of orphans and widows, and the general evisceration of so many nations. I told her about the president of Botswana and the king of

Swaziland who, on separate occasions, and in separate speeches, made the same statement: "If current rates of HIV infection continue without a cure, our nation faces extinction."

I went on to tell her how Kathy and I had become involved in the issue, and of our conviction that a key to combating HIV was a mobilized delivery mechanism of thousands of local churches. I told her about individual churches making a huge difference, and respectfully suggested that any national strategy for Honduras should see the Church as a major player.

"Yes. Yes, I agree," she said. "Now tell me, Pastor, what should I do?"

I was surprised by the candid, child-like, and trusting way in which she asked. I wasn't there to tell her what to do, but here she was, laying her heart on the table and requesting guidance. So, gulping a bit but focused, I began.

"First of all, Donya, you must initiate a major HIV/AIDS awareness campaign for Honduras. You'll need television and newspaper ads, billboards, posters, and whatever else you can use to get a strong, consistent message to your people. They need to know what HIV/AIDS is, how it's contracted, how it can be avoided, and that it is always fatal. Put your face on it. Own it. Let everyone know that this is your issue and you will not rest until HIV/AIDS is defeated.

"Second, you've got to develop a comprehensive educational plan. Focus on children and teens. In fact, in Africa we're starting to talk about HIV/AIDS with kids in Grade One. The average age of sexual activity in Africa is twelve years. This means we've got to get to them before that. We call the under-twelve class the AIDS-free generation. Now, I don't know how you work with your Cabinet, but if I were you, I'd simply instruct your Minister of Education to do whatever is necessary to get a thorough plan together, teach the teachers, and mandate that all Honduran schoolchildren must be HIV/AIDS literate.

"Third, you will have to provide a care and housing infrastructure for children orphaned by AIDS and their widowed mothers. The best care, of course, comes from extended family members. The problem in Africa, however, is that the extended family is overextended. So, think in terms of a major fostering campaign, the construction of small orphan homes, *seven kids per home with a widow as mother figure, and, in cases where it's necessary, orphanages. I know that word is anathema these days, but in Africa there are so many kids falling between the cracks that an orphanage may be the last line of defense. They are certainly a better option than leaving the kids homeless.*

"Finally, you need to think about home-based care for the dying. This is where you'll need an army of volunteers, and this is where the Church can be a huge help. The Church can and should help in the other three areas as well: awareness, education, and housing and care for orphans can all be addressed with great effect by local congregations. But home-based care is something the Church has always done well. We call it visitation. Only now we need to do it with a basin and a towel. And you'll never find a greater pool of committed volunteers than you will in the Church.

"Sound the alarm, Donya. Call the nation to arms. Challenge the Church. Don't take no for an answer. I believe the people will respond. What's more, I believe that the First Ladies of other Central American countries will rally to your cry, as will other nations far away. You may become the spark that ignites a global response. Whatever you do, don't quit. Keep at it. Be faithful. I believe the Lord will be your strength."

I then went on to tell her about the remarkable effect the First Lady of Uganda had had on HIV/AIDS prevalence in her country. How, like Donya, her husband has supported her initiative, and how she had mobilized the women of Uganda in a major assault on the pandemic. I suggested she fly to Uganda and learn from her counterpart personally. And, while she was there, travel to as many other African nations as she could to see what high prevalence means in the faces and the communities of people struck with this awful virus. And, of course, I offered to assist her in any way I could. "We're fellow pilgrims, Donya, and fellow warriors in the greatest war ever to face mankind."

Finally we prayed together, and the meeting ended. But the battle had just begun.

Chapter 4
The Church Stands Up

ddis Ababa, Ethiopia, looks healthy and vibrant when you travel the main streets. Lots of businesses, cars, and street stalls selling everything from candy to DVD players. Lots of people too—some of the most beautiful in the world, I think. But, it's when you get behind the storefronts that it hits you. There, hidden from view, is a rabbit warren of mud-brick hovels and narrow mud streets, so narrow I often had to turn half sideways to pass through. Open sewers, flies, a crush of people, and rampant poverty assault you. In contrast to the relative modernity of the main thoroughfares, the back streets of Addis seem like the dark side of the moon. There is hope, however, in that black hole. A church has lit a flickering candle and the shadows are beginning to flee.

A very large church in Addis had asked me to take a look at their new HIV/AIDS ministry. It also wanted me to spend some time with their leadership. Founded some seventy years ago by the old Sudan Interior Mission, this church now claims a membership of 6 million people. And, from some of the world's poorest people they raise an annual budget of US$36 million!

"How do you do this?" I asked, dumbfounded.

"Everybody tithes," was the straightforward answer. "It doesn't matter if you earn $10 a day or $1 a day. If you're a member of our church, 10 percent of your income belongs to the Lord."

Needless to say, they don't rely on Western financial aid. They fund their comprehensive ministry themselves. Their capacity on every level, whether it is medical care (last year they treated 1 million people for various afflictions) or child advocacy, puts them on the cutting edge in Africa today. As for sustainability, well, as the senior pastor shyly reminded me, "The Christian Church has been in Ethiopia for 1,700 years." Compared to them, the Church in the West is a mere pup.

Before I recount my experience with their home-based care medical team visiting HIV/AIDS sufferers, I need to clarify what I mean when I write about "the Church." I'm not referring to buildings or institutions, nor am I writing about Protestant or Catholic, Orthodox or Charismatic, Eastern or Western, Northern or Southern. I'm writing about people, you and me, in all our shapes, sizes, colors, and varying degrees of piety. For better or for worse, we are the Church. What I'm about to say in this part of the book, I'm taking personally. I hope you will too. But first, let's go to the slums of Addis Ababa.

It's a beautiful Saturday morning in April. I'm walking along a busy street with a doctor and two nurses from the church. They are about to do their rounds. The AIDS patients we're going to see have already been identified, their medical histories have been consulted, and the log is under the arm of the male nurse. This is a serious, professional process and I feel like a bit of a fifth wheel, if not an imposter.

The sights, sounds, and smells of merchant stalls remind me of similar stimuli in so many markets I have visited—the Grand Bazaar in Istanbul, the Shouk in Jerusalem, the Agora in Athens. As we pass one especially vocal fishmonger calling out his special of the day, I wonder how many thousands of merchants are doing the same around the world. Markets have a vitality that reflect the human will to live, eat, drink, consume, and thrive. Caught up in this universal consumer energy, I am blind-sided by a sudden turn past a merchant hawking fake Nikes into a narrow alleyway. It's as though we've jumped from a high platform into dark, forbidding water. We've entered Addis's dark side.

Suddenly everything is a dull brown-gray, the color of sun-baked mud. In other countries where this kind of construction is common, they paint the mud white and call it adobe. Not here. As we walk the uneven dirt alleyways, sometimes turning our upper bodies sideways to avoid jamming our shoulders on the walls, our clothing is soon colored with dust. The farther we walk, the more brown-gray we become.

Another Victim of AIDS

Our first stop is a one-room dwelling (all the dwellings are one room) where a widow lives with her nine-year-old daughter. The mother, who looks to be about twenty-four or twenty-five, is sweeping the floor as we come to the door. She looks up, smiles a brilliant smile, and welcomes us into her very tidy and clean room. The daughter retreats behind her, shyly peeking out at us as we shake hands all around. The doctor, a big, blond American medical missionary from Ohio, pulls out a candy from his pocket and gives it to the little girl, greeting her in fluent Amharic. He introduces me, indulges in a little chit-chat, then gets down to business.

I turn discreetly away as he begins the examination. I hear questions about her diet, her sleep, her diarrhea, and then stand in the doorway looking out onto the sun-baked alley as he places his stethoscope on her bared back and chest to listen for signs of pneumonia. Then as the two Ethiopian nurses take over, he leads the girl out into the sun where I see him casually looking at her arms and legs as he talks to her about last week's Sunday school lesson. I see his face darken with concern.

The nurses complete the log update, we have a quiet word of prayer with this little widow and sweet child, say goodbye, and leave for the next stop. On the way the doctor says, "She's doing better today than she's done lately. She's losing weight, however, and I saw the first signs of oral thrush. But she's got a great attitude. Inspiring really. She could be depressed, but you saw her—she's upbeat, smiling, putting her trust in God." He paused as we rounded a corner and stepped gingerly over an open sewer.

"But the girl?" He shakes his head and sighs.

"What about her?" I ask. "I saw you looking at her skin. Is there a problem?"

"Yes, I think a very serious problem. Looks to me like she's getting shingles, one of the classic signs of stage two AIDS."

"What? I thought you said only the mother was positive."

"I did. But now the girl. I'm afraid that she's been sexually abused."

"Abused?" I was incredulous. "By whom?"

"Oh, it could be an uncle, a cousin, a grandfather, a neighbor, or some stranger. You saw how vulnerable they are. No locks on the door. No one to defend them. Any sexual predator has access." Turning to one of the nurses, he asks her to make a note in the log to inform the social services of his suspicion.

"Will they help?" I ask.

"Not likely," he answers, a note of resignation in his voice. "I mean, they do help in theory, but in practice how do you help her and 10,000 like her just in this area? They're overwhelmed."

"What about the church?" I ask, my stomach hurting with empathy. "Can you do anything?"

"Absolutely. We're caring for their health needs. We are just now preparing a hospice to provide palliative care. We make sure they get proper nutrition. We pray with them. Visit them. But we get overwhelmed too. I wish there were hundreds more churches to help."

Our conversation is interrupted by a passing funeral procession. We flatten ourselves against the wall as one hundred or so grim-faced mourners push past us, a plain wooden coffin leading the way.

"Another victim of AIDS," whispers one of the nurses. "Thousands die every week here in Addis."

We carry on dumbly to our next patient. This one's room has a low tunnel-like corridor forming the narrow part of an "L" leading to a small living area whose walls are covered with religious icons. A heavily perfumed candle burns in a dark red vessel in front of a garish picture of Jesus with an exposed heart. A bed takes up most of the space. There's a small hibachi with live coals providing warmth (and carbon monoxide) for the fevered woman lying in the bed. A ten-year-old girl sits at her feet, her face etched with concern for her mother.

"This one should be in a church hospice," the doctor mutters.

"Why isn't she?" I ask.

"Her priest won't let her. The Ethiopian Church sees us Evangelicals as heretics."

"So why don't they help her?"

"You tell me."

The woman lets out a soul-shaking groan. It's not AIDS that's evoking this, even though she is full-blown.

"It's her shoulder," the doctor explains. "She tried to walk to the toilet last week, fell, and dislocated it. I put it back in place, but she's obviously dislocated it again."

He goes over to the bed, bends down in the semi-darkness, gives her a few instructions, and gently, but firmly, puts the shoulder back in place. She screams with pain. The daughter starts crying. The nurses give comfort, and the doctor fashions a sling out of one of the girl's skirts. He instructs the woman to keep the sling in place. Already she's feeling better. Then he gives her an examination, the log is updated, we pray (at the risk of the priest hearing about it), and we leave. All this in fifteen minutes. And my chest feels like it's going to explode. Compassion can compress your heart to the breaking point. In a whirl we're two doors down, about to enter another darkened room.

This house is obviously owned by someone with a bit more money than the norm. It has a small walled courtyard outside the door. Over in the corner are three foul-smelling vats.

"Take a look," the doctor says.

I go over, remove the cardboard lid of one of the vats, and look at a revolting pus-like scum lying on top of a vile concoction of some sort.

"Gross!" I exclaim.

"It's home brew," says the doctor. "She supplies her neighborhood men with drink. She used to sell her body. Now she sells her brew."

We're met at the door by a tall, thin woman who, even in her AIDS-afflicted state, has a haunting presence and beauty. We go into her room and, after some small talk, the examination begins.

The doctor begins with her mouth. As she opens it I'm shocked by what I see. The lining is covered with a rough white coating that, according to the examination, extends deep down into her esophagus. She sits passively and expressionless on a low backless stool as the nurses apply a topical cream. While this is going on I happen to look up at a picture of Sophia Loren on the wall.

"Why would she have a movie star on her wall?" I wonder to myself. Then it hits me. It's not Sophia Loren, it's her! I look down, the nurses finished with their task, and ask, "Is that you?" She smiles faintly and nods.

"Yes, it's me. In my former days." Her voice is weak, her English impeccable.

I turn away as the examination continues, not just for discretion's sake, but to hide my tears. On our way, after prayer, the doctor says,

"The esophageal thrush is a bad sign. She's entering stage four. I don't expect she'll live much longer."

"She was so beautiful," I say.

"Yes. Still is."

We walk in silence, our senses dulled to the squalor around us. We duck under some laundry hanging across the alley and enter a small square with a tree growing in the middle. Just past the tree is a faded yellow door.

We duck as we enter yet another darkened room. A bed takes up a third of the space; at the back behind a curtain is a closet kitchen. A young woman lies in the bed. Another young woman sits at the end of it. Standing around it are a young man and an older woman, dressed immaculately. The doctor knows them all.

The young woman in the bed is seventeen and has full-blown AIDS. Her friend sitting at the end is also seventeen, and has early onset AIDS. Her skin is beginning to show signs of shingles. Her name is Jerusalem. The older woman (who is only thirty-five) is HIV negative, but has been suffering from a horrible female affliction since delivering her first baby twenty-two years ago. It's called a fistula. And the young man—well, he's HIV positive and is a defrocked preacher. His denomination withdrew his credentials when his status was revealed. Now, without home or income, he ministers daily to the AIDS sufferers of Addis, sleeping wherever and eating whatever the Lord provides. He looks good.

We've interrupted a prayer meeting. The girl in the bed was too weak to come to the meeting, so the meeting has come to her. The examination of all four and the updating of the log take about forty minutes.

As the doctor and nurses repack their bags, Jerusalem says, "We were about to pray when you arrived. Would you stay and pray with us?" As someone who cut his teeth on a church pew and who has attended thousands of church and prayer meetings over the years, you'll understand me when I say this was the first prayer meeting I've ever attended.

All four lift their hands and voices to heaven. There is no preamble, no setting the stage, no windup. They simply transfer their focus from this world to the other. Indeed, one senses that they are already more in synch with heaven than earth. They pray with intensity, sincerity, power. I feel like the Presence is descending upon us. It pushes me down. There is such a sense of the holy. I want to prostrate myself, confess my sins, or get out of there. But at that moment, all but the girl in the bed come over, lay their hands on me, and begin to pray for "Pasta Jim."

So here are people with their feet in the grave, acquainted with suffering and grief, marginalized by their friends and neighbors, with every reason to be angry and bitter, lifting me up before the Almighty. I was prayed for by fifteen pastors at my ordination, I've been prayed for by various congregants at critical decision points in my years of pastoring, and I've received numerous letters and e-mails from viewers of my television shows telling me they're praying for me. Yes, I've been prayed for, but never like this. It's as though they've taken me by the hand into the very throne room of God. There, they're trying to convince the Creator that "Pasta Jim" is a good man, doing a much needed but unpopular ministry, championing the cause of orphans and widows, critical to the future of Africa and the world. You can understand how I'm feeling. "No Lord, that's not me. I'm just a water boy, a servant. A tool in your hand. They're overstating it, Lord. No. No. I've got to get out of here. I can't take this. I'm so unworthy." But my feet are rooted to the floor. I can't move.

When the prayers end, I walk out into the sunshine in a daze. I can't speak, nor do I want to. I want nothing to break the spell. I'm totally at peace. I've been in the presence of the King.

Once again I'm reminded of a gripping reality that I confront everywhere in Africa. The Africans are so materially poor, yet so spiritually rich. We Westerners, on the other hand, are very rich materially, but we're so spiritually poor. Could it be that as we reach out to alleviate their material poverty, they reach back to alleviate our spiritual poverty? If that's the case, it's certainly not intentional, at least on the Africans' part. But it's simply true that if you are kind to the poor, the poor are kind to you. Sometimes you wonder who is helping whom.

The best-case scenario occurs when Africans help Africans. This is what is happening in Addis. And it's starting to happen throughout Africa. As I see it, the African Church is the champion that can break the back of HIV/AIDS and emerge as a "father to the fatherless and defender of widows."

Rather than stand back and watch, the Church in the West needs to be engaged at this vital time. We have so much that can truly help the African Church do its work. If we go in, not as conquerors or coloniz-ers, but as servants, giving the Africans our time, talent, and treasure, we'll discover a powerful win–win relationship that will add huge value on both sides of the Atlantic. What's more, it will see us sensitized and activated with regard to our own poor. Rather than a culture of service receivers, we'll become a culture of service providers. No longer will we ask the question, "Is our Church relevant to the culture?" Instead, we'll know the real question is, "Is our Church relevant to the poor?"

In the last chapter, I examined the essential DNA of the biblical view of God's opposition to injustice and his prior commitment to the "alien, the orphan and the widow." Now I want to look at the Church as God's hand extended to the poor. We've got to get off the sidelines and into the game. HIV/AIDS is forcing us out of our comfort zone. The millions of orphans and widows are crying out for a defender. The Church must respond proactively with faith, hope, and love. *It is time for the Church to stand up.*

Faith: Where We Begin

My Jerusalem lawyer said he had never laughed so much over anything related to his practice. "You remember, Jim," he laughed, his eyes spar-kling, "that time you and the rabbi signed the contract?"

"I do, I do," I said, laughing too.

"Upon the event of messiah coming to Jerusalem, Cantelon agrees to vacate the premises within the month." Uproarious laughter. Through tears of hilarity he continued, "That clause I've never seen before. I'm sure in all the history of negotiation in Israel those words have never been included in a contract. Ha! Ha! Can you believe it?"

"But he was serious," I added. "Totally serious."

He was pleased to rent the flat to me—in fact, I think it tickled him to rent to a "Christian Zionist," as he called me, but he sure wanted to guarantee my departure should the messiah show up. He said he'd bought the place for that eventuality. "As soon as the messiah comes," he said, "I'm moving from Toronto to Jerusalem." The rabbi was ortho-dox, and his faith, indeed his life, was predicated on the hope that he would live to see and participate in the messianic era. But until then, let the gentile pay the mortgage!

James, Jesus's half-brother, was orthodox too. Indeed he was ultra-orthodox, so pious that even though he was the head of the Church in Jerusalem, no one could find fault with him. Tradition tells us he used to go up to the temple every day—that would have been about two hundred steps—on his knees! He lived a kosher life, was adamant in his insistence that he and all believers should keep the law, and, to all appearances, was a Jew of the Jews. He was spiritually mature, and very keen to discuss, preach, teach, or communicate in any way the true meaning of faith. Fortunately for us, he put his thoughts and beliefs in writing. The document appears in the New Testament. It's called the Book of James.

A Christian response to AIDS in Africa has got to begin with faith, not religion. Religion is so fraught with mini- and subcultures that we often tend to be defensive. Proving "who is right" takes all our energy. No. We've got to get beyond our interpretive filters of the scriptures. We've got to understand faith. We've got to practise it. We've got to live it because the Bible itself says, "without faith it is impossible to please God" (Heb. 11:6). James helps us know what it is, and how to make it work.

James has often been viewed as a contrarian because of his coun-terculture view of wealth and poverty. For us, and for most everyone else throughout history, wealth is the reward for diligence, hard work, and business acumen. We see it as a blessing from God, something to be celebrated, something to aspire to, and the rich are to be emulated. It is "wise" to accumulate wealth, "prudent" to provide for one's old age (the more affluent, the better), and it's "the American way." Lots of money is good. Little money is bad. Poverty is a curse. Even a little boasting is appropriate for the rich—if not in words, then in the size of one's home, the beam of one's sailboat, or the fitness of one's body. The poor, on the other hand, shrink into the shadows. Nobody wants to be poor.

So, what does James say? "Believers who are poor have something to boast about, for God has honored them. And those who are rich should boast that God has humbled them" (1:9, 10). I must admit that I have found these words disturbing and unsettling over the years. It's not my nature to absorb guilt, but I found these words laying on guilt in a very definite "in your face" kind of way. I found myself justifying materialistic tendencies, excusing discontent with my relative "poverty," defending the desire to be rich and carefree. And, when I read the rest of what he says about poverty and riches, my eyes glazed over with defensive irritation. "He can't be serious," I reasoned. And frankly, if it weren't for my exposure to suffering orphans and widows in Africa over the past few years, I'm sure I would still be offended by James' harshness.

Now I can understand James' point when he says, "Hasn't God chosen the poor in this world to be rich in faith? Aren't they the ones who will inherit the kingdom He promised to those who love him?" (2:5). The African orphans and widows with whom I have interacted have taught me the truth of this scripture. The Ethiopian prayer meeting is a case in point. There's no doubt in my mind that in that powerful moment of intercession I was merely a child, a naif, and they were the ones who knew the way—in some parallel-universe sense they were leading me into what for them was familiar territory. The "Kingdom" was their homeland. And, with the generosity of spirit that exists only for those lacking arrogance, they were kindly introducing me to the King.

I think of something the prophet Jeremiah said to the wise, the strong, and the rich in Judah:

> [23]This is what the Lord says: "Let not the wise man boast of his wisdom or the strong man boast of his strength or the rich man boast of his riches,
>
> [24]but let him who boasts boast about this: that he understands and knows me, that I am the Lord, who exercises kindness, justice and righteousness on earth, for in these I delight," declares the Lord. (9:23, 24)

It seems that a biblical faith puts us at odds with our world's values. Faith is counterculture in that it appeals to and lives within the context of an expectation of supernatural intervention and authority.

It relies not on self but on Other; it stresses dependence rather than independence. Money is eclipsed by "un-money." Indeed, heaven provides a powerful commentary by paving its roads with what our world considers to be the most precious of resources: gold. Our riches are heaven's tar pits. Little wonder then that history's saints were not motivated by money. They had their eyes on a greater prize.

James assumes that riches are achieved unjustly:

> **5** Look here, you rich people, weep and groan with anguish because of all the terrible troubles ahead of you. ²Your wealth is rotting away, and your fine clothes are moth-eaten rags. ³Your gold and silver have become worthless. The very wealth you were counting on will eat away your flesh in hell. This treasure you have accumulated will stand as evidence against you on the day of judgment. ⁴For listen! Hear the cries of the field workers whom you have cheated of their pay. The wages you held back cry out against you. The cries of the reapers have reached the ears of the Lord Almighty.
>
> ⁵You have spent your years on earth in luxury, satisfying your every whim. Now your hearts are nice and fat, ready for the slaughter. ⁶You have condemned and killed good people who had no power to defend themselves against you. (5:1–5)

Perhaps in his day this was true. It's certainly true today in many of Africa's "kleptocracies" where brutally self-indulgent leaders are building their offshore bank accounts on the backs of their beleaguered peasants. Perhaps the closest any of us can come to wealth via injustice is our willingness to look the other way as the manufacturers of so many of our goods exploit the sweatshops of China in pursuit of higher profits. No one's hands, including mine, are clean.

The Far Country

Several years ago, after days of intensive on-camera work for a national television show in Australia, my crew and I took a break and drove up to the Gold Coast, north of Sydney, for a day at the beach. We stopped at a beautiful spot popular with surfers, and watched in awe as young people rode huge swells that became 20-foot monster waves as they broke toward the shore. When they ended each run, some gracefully, others indecorously, they lay prone on their boards, paddled over to a certain spot, and were whisked back out to sea, as if they were on one of those moving sidewalks we see at airports. I commented on this, and one of my Aussie crew said, "They're riding the riptide."

"What's a riptide?" I asked.

"Well, all that water crashing up on the beach has got to exit somewhere, so it exits in rivers back out to the depths."

"Rivers?"

"Yeah, you know, like underwater currents. They're so powerful that if a swimmer gets caught in one, we've learned not to fight it but to ride it until it loses its grip. Fight it and you drown."

James is warning us about the riptide of riches. You can use money or it uses you. As a commodity for redemptive purposes, money can be a great thing. But if it's seen as a means to personal aggrandizement, or as a substitute for dependence on the Creator, it can be a bad thing.

Dependence is the issue. The Bible makes it clear that the Almighty wants to be the Almighty. He wants us to be in need of his might. That's why Jesus said we're to be like little children. Kids start out dependent, but as they grow, their desire for independence grows too. As adults, we need to understand that worldliness is independence. We want to be our own source and beginning, our own provider, our own final court of appeal. We don't want to need God, or others for that matter, for anything. If we're religious, we give God the glory for our independence—we spiritualize our self-sufficiency. So we protect ourselves from vulnerability; we flee exposure to poverty, disease, and decay. We turn away from the marginalized, for in the eyes of the poor, we see our own vulnerability staring back at us. We don't want this. We want to be financially secure, healthy, and immune to "the slings and arrows of outrageous fortune." We want to retreat behind our retirement savings and pretend that we can cheat death.

If this sounds harsh, how do we get around the words, "This treasure you have accumulated will stand as evidence against you on the day of judgment"? Yes, I know most of us have not accumulated our material possessions by cheating our employees or misusing the courts to condemn and kill innocent people, but we've got to see what James sees here. He sees space and time as merely the gate to the Kingdom of Heaven. Somehow we're determining the DNA of our spiritual character here on earth that will not be fully expressed until we become the planting of the Lord in the eternities. How we live now, the values we embrace, the relationships we cultivate with God and neighbor, are all critical components of our future capacity to flourish in the Kingdom of Heaven. James sees independence as a killer. We've got to be childlike in our faith, depending on no one but our heavenly father. And one way or another, the Almighty sees to it that we remain dependent. Often the meaning behind some of life's accidents is found in a loving heavenly father keeping us keenly aware of where our true strength lies.

In James's view, poverty leads positively to honor, riches negatively to humility, which is a good thing in both cases, especially as it is God who both honors and humbles. But the point is this: socioeconomic status in this world means nothing in the world to come. And if you've been honored and/or humbled by God, then you qualify to enter his Kingdom as a citizen. As James sees it, life is all about "the far country."

Which brings us to faith—what is it? Let's read what James says:

> [14]*What good is it, dear brothers and sisters, if you say you have faith but don't show it by your actions? Can that kind of faith save anyone?* [15]*Suppose you see a brother or a sister who has no food or clothing,* [16]*and you say, "Good-bye and have a good day; stay warm and eat well"—but then you don't give that person any food or clothing. What good does that do?*
>
> [17]*So you see, faith by itself isn't enough. Unless it produces good deeds, it is dead and useless. (2:14–17)*

These words are bookended by two observations that require some consideration before addressing what faith is. They both are abuses of Christianity. The first is:

> [8] *... it is good when you obey the royal law as found in the Scriptures: "love your neighbor as yourself." [9] But if you favor some people over others, you are committing a sin. You are guilty of breaking the law. (2:8, 9)*

And the second:

> [19] *You say you have faith, for you believe that there is one God. Good for you! Even the demons believe this, and they tremble in terror. [20] How foolish! Can't you see that faith without good deeds is useless? (2:19, 20)*

The first abuse is discrimination in favor of the rich rationalized as obedience to "the royal law." The second is verbal righteousness hiding behind the skirts of monotheism. In other words, discriminatory justice and passive righteousness won't cut it. A monotheistic faith without action is "mono-useless." Or, as Soren Kierkegaard once said, "Mere mental assent to a doctrine is not enough. Where there is no transformation there is no Christianity." Faith and action, righteousness and justice, are like "love and marriage" or "a horse and carriage"—you can't have one without the other.

So what is faith? Faith, as James argues, is action. Look at 2:14–17 again. Inactive faith has no supernatural linkage. It can't "save anyone" (v. 14). Regardless of piety, fervency, or religiosity, a faith that is immune to the suffering of a brother or sister is both useless and a mockery. It has no life because it has no soul. It reeks of self-indulgence and self-deception. It's a "form of godliness," but denies "the power thereof" (2 Tim. 3:5, KJV). Without breath, the body is dead.

I might put it this way: Right belief plus right action equals faith. Or, righteousness plus justice equals faith. Or, R + J = F. The point is, if you're going to be a person of faith, you've got to be a player. Spectators need not apply.

The classic comment from James, of course, is his word about "pure and genuine religion" in 1:27. It's a powerful sentence that captures R + J = F: "Pure and genuine religion in the sight of God the Father means caring for orphans and widows in their distress and refusing to let the world corrupt you."

Notice there's nothing about piety, ritual, or tradition here. Nothing about systems, methodologies, or cultural relevance. Not a word about sincerity. Rather, a high view of neighbor (care for the orphan and widow) coupled with a high view of God (unworldliness) will see one acting in such a way that one is purely and genuinely religious. Evil flees in the face of true love for God and neighbor.

This supernaturally sparked and empowered love for God and neighbor elevates what could be seen as mere philanthropy to pure religion. We're not talking about "do good, feel good" here. We're way above altruism as well. What we're talking about is the Church—the Body of Christ—extending an arm to the orphan and widow that in every sense breaks through the divide between heaven and earth. Our care means God's care. We're the only Jesus the orphan and widow will ever see on planet earth. Our love for them is both rooted and generated in the very heart of God himself. True religion is God come down in us.

Hope: The Engine of Faith

The writer of the book of Hebrews might look at the R + J = F equation and remark that something is missing. He'd probably add "hope" and draw it this way:

$$\frac{R + J}{H} = F$$

Let me explain: "Faith is the substance of things hoped for the evidence of things not seen" (KJV).

This is the opening sentence of the famous Chapter 11, which is usually called "the great faith chapter." It's a marvelous account of several biblical characters who were men and women of action. Not content with settling their lives around a passive confession of monotheism, they struck their tents and headed out to the far horizon, "not knowing whither they went." They were righteous and just, true heroes of faith, and their actions changed the world.

The question the writer answers is: What motivated them? Was it the need for adventure? A search for new pastures? Discontent with the status quo? Great love for God and neighbor? Nomadic DNA? Was it all of the above, or none of it? The writer answers by saying they did what they did "by faith." In fact, "by faith" occurs twenty-three times in the course of forty verses. But he doesn't describe faith as James does. Faith is predicated on more than law and duty in his view. He sees the great catalyst for faith action to be vision, or "hope"—the "unseen" provides the undercurrent for great acts of righteousness and justice. The heroes of faith would never have been heroes without it.

I chose to quote the King James version because of the strong words: "substance ... things hoped for ... evidence ... things not seen." Here you have something clearly visible predicated on and indicative of something totally invisible. Like James, the writer sees faith as action, and its motivation is unseen but vitally there. Just as the wind is unseen but powerful, so too hope is insubstantial but capable of transforming glowing embers into a raging firestorm.

If the Church is going to stand up and face the HIV/AIDS pandemic head on, we will have to do more than care for its victims. We will have to give a stricken continent hope for the future. To do that we've got to understand the key role that hope plays in active faith. Hebrews, Chapter 11, needs to be inculcated into the very heart of who we are, so let's take some time and digest this classic.

First of all, a word about the book of Hebrews itself. The writer (unknown to us—some call him or her "the preacher") is writing to Jewish believers who have dispersed into the various countries around the Mediterranean ocean. They have grown weary of persecution and frustrated that the gospel they bought into has let them down. The messiah has not returned. They figure they've been duped, so many are "forsaking the assembling of themselves together" and are going back to their former reliance on blood sacrifice as a means of atonement for sin. So the writer writes to remind them not only of the fervency of their faith in earlier days, but also about the superiority of Christ's sacrifice and the hope for the future it brings:

> [32] *Don't ever forget those early days when you first learned about Christ. Remember how you remained faithful even though it meant terrible suffering.*
>
> [33] *Sometimes you were exposed to public ridicule and were beaten, and sometimes you helped others who were suffering the same things.*
>
> [34] *You suffered along with those who were thrown into jail. When all you owned was taken from you, you accepted it with joy. You knew you had better things waiting for you in eternity.*
>
> [35] *Do not throw away this confident trust in the Lord, no matter what happens. Remember the great reward it brings you!*
>
> [36] *Patient endurance is what you need now, so you will continue to do God's will. Then you will receive all that he has promised.*
>
> [37] *"For in just a little while, the Coming One will come and not delay.*
>
> [38] *And a righteous person will live by faith. But I will have no pleasure in anyone who turns away."*
>
> [39] *But we are not like those who turn their backs on God and seal their fate. We have faith that assures our salvation. (10:32–39)*

The hope the writer underscores is in an unseen God, an elusive messiah, and an unseen "country they can call their own" (11:14). Active faith is all about hope, says the preacher. In Chapter 11 he preaches hard.

A Gentile in a Jewish Pulpit

I've preached over 4,000 times in my ministry career—that's a lot of sermons and a lot of pulpit time. One of my most enduring memories of a sermon and a pulpit is of the time I was invited to preach at a conservative synagogue in Toronto. It was the summer of 1982, and Israel had recently invaded Lebanon.

Disturbing reports in the media had upset the Jewish community worldwide. Reports of atrocities and human rights abuses by the Israeli army against the Lebanese populace abounded. I knew many of these reports were spurious, cobbled together by journalists from second- and third-hand information. I could understand this because I myself had witnessed their frustration as they gathered from all over the world at the Arazim Hotel in Metulla, Israel's northernmost town, right on the border with Lebanon. Each time I returned to Metulla from my broadcasting post in southern Lebanon, the journalists would cluster around probing me for information. They wanted to check the veracity of what they had heard from various sources. Not allowed by Israel to enter the invasion zone, they were an angry and milling mob of disgruntlement. One of them even tried to bribe me, asking that I hide him in the trunk of my car as I drove through the Fatima Gate into the restricted area. At that time I was one of three foreigners in northern Israel with a military pass. I was also one of the few able to give a first-hand account of what was truly happening.

This was why a synagogue had a gentile in the pulpit. They asked me to preach (from Genesis) and to include a report on what I had seen in Tyre, Sidon, and the region around Khleia and Marjayoun. They wanted me to bear witness to what I had seen, to paint a picture of what they hadn't seen. They needed some substance, some evidence enabling them to understand what was going on so far away.

I stood in their beautiful pulpit, my shoulders draped in a graceful *talith* (prayer shawl), my head covered with a *kippa* (skullcap). Looking down at 600 grim-faced Jews, I began:

> I'm here today because your faith in Israel has been shaken. Mine would be too if all we had to go on was the newspaper and television reports. I'm here to tell you what I have seen with my own eyes over the past few months in Lebanon. I'm also here to expose some of Genesis to you. But before I do either, let me take a moment and ask, "What is faith"?
>
> One of the writers of the New Testament, writing to the Hebrews, says this: "Now faith is the substance of things hoped for, the evidence of things not seen." Sounds ambiguous, but let me try to bring some clarity to the ideas.

I think this beautiful pulpit in which I'm standing is made of oak. It is in great condition, especially in that your rabbi tells me it's over 100 years old. It's very substantial, and it's evidence of so much we can't see. For instance, it is evidence that perhaps two or three hundred years ago an acorn fell to the ground somewhere in North America, and, against all odds, germinated and took root. It is evidence that it withstood decades of hot summers, cold winters, storms, and forest fires. It also avoided being eaten by wildlife or being uprooted by someone looking to transplant a young oak to their garden. Slowly it grew while other less substantial trees took root, grew, and died. Over decades it became the king of its patch of forest. But, one day a logging surveyor came along, looked at its bulk and height, and made a note for the tree cutters. This pulpit is evidence that the tree was cut down, taken to a mill, and cut into lumber. It is also evidence that someone studied cabinetry and fine-furniture making. It is evidence that this cabinet maker decided to accept a commission from the local synagogue to build a pulpit. It is evidence that the rabbi had a design in mind, and the cabinet maker the skill to make the design a wondrous work in wood. It is evidence that thousands of sermons have been preached from it, and hundreds of cantors have sung from it. It is also evidence that hundreds more sermons, songs, and services will see it standing here majestically in the future. Yes, this pulpit is "the substance, and the evidence, of all kinds of things we cannot see."

Let me stop, lest I preach a sermon here. The point is clear, however: faith is substantial, evidential—it's the product of an unseen past and unseen future, and the action in the present of a visionary who sees both. That product is often the action itself, but there's nothing if there's not vision first. Faith simply makes the dream come true. Or, to put it another way, faith is the body, hope the soul.

This chapter of Hebrews (11) reads like an overview of Israel's early history. It recounts the motivation of several heroes such as Abel, Enoch, Noah, Abraham, Sarah, Isaac, Jacob, Moses, Rahab, and many unnamed martyrs. That motivation? Hope. Their faith actions were contingent on seeing the unseen.

For example, look at Noah. He is warned by God "about things that had never happened before" (v. 7) and, on the basis of that warning does something that's never been done before. He builds an ark (What's an ark?) to save his family from the flood (What's a flood?). It takes several years to build (some commentators suggest 120 years!) and, as he builds, he warns people about something that he hasn't seen. They laugh, shrug, cluck their tongues at this madman, express sympathy for his wife, and carry on. In every sense of the word, Noah's ark was his faith. It was the substance, the evidence of something he hadn't seen as yet. It was the personification, or should I say "arkification" of his hope.

Or take Abraham. He moves his considerable household from Ur (modern-day southern Iraq) up to Haran (modern-day Syria) by foot—a huge undertaking through almost impassable desert mountains. Sarah is just getting her kitchen tent in order when Abraham walks in with that faraway look in his eye.

"Oh no!" she thinks. Abraham plops himself down on the richly carpeted floor and clears his throat.

"Sarah, we're going to move."

"What? Move! We just got here!"

"I know, I know, but the Lord has told me we're to move again."

"I can't believe this," Sarah mutters, thinking maybe her husband has spent too much time in the sun with the goats. "So, where are we going?"

"Well, uh, that's just the point. I'm, uh, not sure where we're going."

"You're not sure?" she responds, a touch of disgust in her voice. "You're not sure? So, what are you looking for? You've got to know that at least."

"Actually, um, I'm, uh, looking for a city that's not there."

We'll leave Sarah to her mutterings. The writer tells us Abraham "was confidently looking forward to a city with eternal foundations, a city designed and built by God" (v. 10). He was looking for the heavenly Jerusalem—a city, by the way, that's still not there. On the basis of something he hadn't seen as yet, Abraham, like Noah, acted differently than anyone else of his generation. In every sense of the word, Abraham's trek from Ur to Haran and down to Shechem was his faith.

It was the substance, the evidence, of something invisible. It was the "trekification" of his hope.

Then there's Abraham and Sarah. He's 100 years old, she's 90. Even in their long-living era she was past childbearing years. One evening Abraham comes home with some wildflowers he's picked for her. He lights a few candles, why, he's even sweetened his breath. And he has that twinkle in his eye. Sarah can't believe it.

"Abraham! Forget it. We're old, you know. Very old. I love you for sure, but sex at our age? Come on, Abraham. Leave it to the young."

"But, Sarah. Have you forgotten? God has promised us a son. Remember? He's going to make of us a great nation. God has promised."

"Great faith you've got," she says, turning away.

Abraham comes up behind her, folds his arms around her, and whispers, "Yes, great faith, but faith without works is dead!" Nine months later Isaac is born.

On the basis of something they hadn't seen as yet, Abraham and Sarah acted differently than any other 100-year-old couple in their neighborhood. In every sense of the word, their act of sex was their faith. It was the "sexualization" of their hope.

The writer points out that all these heroes of faith were motivated by hope; they came to a God they couldn't see (v. 6), they set out on journeys not knowing their destination (v. 8), they died pursuing hope that was unfulfilled (v. 13), and were content to spend their lives chasing a dream that was always at a distance (v. 13b). Indeed, every one of them, known and unknown, predicated their lives on a "hope in a better life after the resurrection" (v. 35). That is why "God is not ashamed to be called their God, for he has prepared a city for them" (v. 16).

Heroes of Hope

One cool winter's day Kathy and I were guests at a church service in Mwanza, Tanzania. The city is beautifully situated on the shore of Lake Victoria, but it is far from beautiful. It is full of squat, well-worn little shops, dirt roads (badly potholed), cows, goats, and throngs of people buying, selling, and begging. Perhaps its most remarkable feature, however, is the terrain upon which it is built. Climbing up from the shore of the lake to great heights above are massive stone outcroppings that look like the artwork of some tribe of giants. It's as if they decided to have a contest to see who could pile the most boulders in the most complex way, with a premium on making the piles look as precarious as possible. The boulders, by the way, are humongous stones anywhere from 20 to 100 feet in diameter! In, among, and on top of these natural wonders sit the humble homes of the Mwanzans. They look so vulnerable. I remember one house built right up against a huge boulder of about 70 feet in diameter, towering above. It looked like it was ready to roll down to the lake, crushing everything, including this little hovel, in its path. But the woman of the house was hanging up laundry, totally oblivious to the hulking threat—just another day in paradise. Her home, by the way, was only a few steps from the church.

The church building was perched on top of one of these giant sculptures. To get to it we had to climb a well-worn path through the boulders to oversized, out-of-camber cement steps leading up to the out-of-plumb doorway. Indeed, the entire building, humble and well worn, looked out of plumb. It seemed as if it had slid into place from a higher plane, and had settled in its present location, arrested by a huge rock. It wasn't going anywhere, but leaned forward as if it were looking at a far horizon. And, even though there were no truly vertical or horizontal lines in the entire edifice, it looked solid and well grounded. It had the bearing of a rock itself.

We had to take a big step up into the building. It took a moment for our eyes to adjust to the dimness. The only light was soft, slanting through narrow slits in the walls, falling gently on backless benches and a small congregation of about thirty women, twenty children, five babies, and six men. The floor was uneven and continued climbing right up to the front where we sat in the seat of honor, two chairs with backs, right at the foot of a rough-hewn cross anchored with seven small boulders.

The pastor opened the service with a humble prayer, and then the congregation began to sing. Kathy and I have been in scores of African church services over the years, but we're always in awe of the Africans' superior gift for expressing praise to God in music. Quite simply, they are the best. Other cultures open their mouths to sing; Africans open their souls. Everything moves. Everything vibrates. It's as though an ocean current is flowing over soft coral and every fiber of that underwater world comes alive. Flashes of gold, brilliant blue, and silver cascade through the coral as schools of tiny fish feed on the microscopic life riding the current. The larger parrotfish and angelfish, stunning in their primal colors, feed on the hard coral and occasionally on the smaller fish. The eels and groupers, deeper and lurking in the shadows, lend their sober, stabilizing presence, and the overall feeling of the swimmer, mask, snorkel, and fins giving him access to this parallel universe, is one of quiet and awe. One has intruded upon a mystic world of purity and wholeness. Bathed in the filtered light of the reef, or the sacred light of the humble church, one treads lightly. The Holy One is here. Heaven listens when an African church sings.

As our souls bathe in this cleansing stream, I take a few steps to the side wall, turn, and look at this human pipe organ. The women wear bright, multicolored dresses, the men dark pants and white shirts. The children wear shorts and T-shirts. Everyone looks clean and cared for. Their faces are all turned heavenward, their eyes closed, their hands raised and waving, their bodies moving as one to the rhythm of a haunting Swahili melody. Some of the children stand on and a few kneel on the benches, faces fast to the rough wooden planking. No one looks around. There is total focus here. Total soul. Total love for a God they cannot see.

The thing is, they've nothing to sing about or praise God for. They're poor. Some are sick. One or two appear to be victims of "the slim disease." I see skin lesions, and one woman, as she sings, opens her mouth to reveal thrush. They should be despairing, not praising. Their songs should be a dirge, not an anthem of worship. What's going on here?

Hope is going on here. These are heroes of faith who have seen a far country and have set their hearts on dwelling there. Their sufferings are just for the moment. Death will be a release, for they "place their hope in a better life after the resurrection." This is why they sing of "Jesu" ("Jesus" in Swahili). He has borne their sufferings. He has taken their sin upon himself and has died so they might live. He has risen from the dead, proving once and for all not just the legitimacy of his claim to divinity, but also becoming "the first fruits of them that shall also rise." He is their savior, their healer, their comforter, their never-failing friend. In him "they live, and move, and have their being." He is their hope, their light in a dark place.

This light is everywhere in Africa. But generally it is hiding under a bushel, covered over by major denial as far as HIV/AIDS is concerned. There is huge potential for the churches in Africa to be a continent-wide delivery mechanism for HIV/AIDS proactivity. They just have to be awakened. We don't need to bring hope from the West. All we need to bring is a trumpet call to action. There's more than enough hope to go around.

So, let the African Church stand up. If hope is the key to faith action, then the Church is Africa's strongest and brightest light. Let it shine. Let HIV/AIDS, like the darkness, flee in the face of an awakened Church.

Love of Neighbor: The True Fix for a Better World

It had been a dark and stormy night. In the early morning light, the rain continued to fall. I stole quietly from our bed, leaving Kathy covered from head to foot in the goose-down duvet (only her nose and one big toe exposed—a favorite sleeping posture of hers!), and quickly put on my rain gear. I was going out into the rain to walk. Walking is one of the joys of my life, especially in early morning rain. I love the solitude, too. I relished the chance to enjoy wet solitude for an hour or so. There was a distinct spring in my step as I set out. I didn't know I'd return with a powerful picture forever etched on my mind.

Our neighborhood bordered on the countryside, so as I walked I saw and heard the birds, soaked and ruffled though they were, flitting about and loudly declaring their lordship of territory. I also saw a be-draggled fox quickly leaping into the woods at my approach. I turned down a lane that was more a tunnel than a walkway because it was totally canopied by tall maples, and reveled in the stillness. At the far end was a large park, beautifully maintained and, at this time of the morning, totally empty, and totally mine.

Some thoughtful town father had convinced the park authorities to construct a long sidewalk that cut diagonally from corner to corner of the vast expanse of lawn, so as I entered the park, I took to this ribbon of cement. But then I hesitated and stopped.

The sidewalk was covered in dew worms. You know, those big fat worms that surface during a heavy downpour to avoid drowning—the ones that fishermen pay a lot for. They're big, juicy, and the goal of all those robins hop-hop-hopping around, their heads cocked, their beaks slashing at the ground, was to capture and swallow them whole. Well, the rain had been so intense overnight that the lawns were totally soaked, with puddles of standing water everywhere. So, the dew worms, no fools, had migrated to higher ground—in this case, the sidewalk. There they lay, relatively immobile, a veritable smorgasbord for robins.

I was amazed, as I gingerly stepped over worm after worm, at the scores of robins ignoring the fast food and continuing their hop-and-seize ritual on the grass. They were having a very difficult time because most of the lawn was covered with standing water. And, on those higher patches of grass, there were no worms to be found. They'd all migrated.

"Hey guys. Over here!" I spoke out loud to the eager hunters. "Look! Can't you see? They're all here on the sidewalk! Over here, guys."

Not one responded. They were too intensely focused on doing it the way they'd always done it. They were stuck in their ways. There was only one way to catch a worm. And nobody, especially a human, was going to tell them how to do it.

"What a waste," I thought as I stood in the middle of the park, surrounded by mist, inert, stranded worms, and bobbing robins. "When the sun comes up they'll start to die, and the robins will keep on hopping and pecking. Here's a feast they could tell their grandbirds about, but they don't even see it." And then I thought of the Church, hopping and pecking away, pursuing her programmed ways, totally oblivious to the inert and stranded souls under her nose. Content with maintaining her proven subculture of "faith," happy to navel-gaze, satisfied to embrace those who embrace her, preferring the sentimental to the sacred, she marches on, sure of herself and certain of a warm welcome on the other side. As for the poor generally, or the victims of HIV/AIDS specifically, "Huh? Where are they? I haven't seen any poor people in our church. And, frankly, Jim, the poor are poor for a reason. You know, they need a work ethic. And as far as those AIDS people are concerned, well, I wouldn't want to say this publicly, but, hey, Jim, they're only getting what they deserve. Don't quote me on that, but you know what I mean." And she bobs along, the champion of conditional love. But:

> **13** *If I could speak all the languages of earth and of angels, but didn't love others, I would only be a noisy gong or a clanging cymbal. ²If I had the gift of prophecy, and if I understood all of God's secret plans and possessed all knowledge, and if I had such faith that I could move mountains, but didn't love others, I would be nothing. ³If I gave everything I have to the poor and even sacrificed my body, I could boast about it, but if I didn't love others, I would have gained nothing. (1 Cor. 13:1–3)*

The scriptures make it clear that the Almighty is the champion of unconditional love. The word for love in this famous chapter is *agape*, which refers generally to the undeserved grace we have received from God. It cannot be returned to him apart from our loving our neighbor. If we're going to sing the old hymn "More love to thee, O Christ," we've got to follow quickly with "Rescue the Perishing." To fulfill the demands of righteousness, one must love one's neighbor. Indeed, as the scripture says, "If we don't love people we can see, how can we love God, whom we cannot see?" (1 Jn. 4:20b). *Agape* says, "Okay, you've freely received love you don't deserve from God. To show you're grateful, do the same for your neighbor." This is why righteousness and justice can be fulfilled only through love. Love for God (righteousness) means love for neighbor (justice). A god-seeker is a justice-seeker. With no conditions.

As I write I've just returned from Charlotte, North Carolina, where I attended the longest Nascar race in North America, the Coca-Cola 600. Held at the Lowes Motor Speedway in Concord, it is 600 miles of ear-shattering fury. Stock cars hurtle around the mile-and-a-half track at speeds approaching 200 miles an hour. They roar, growl, screech, and thunder past the grandstands, bits of dirt and rubber literally impacting the 150,000 fans, the sound so loud that it can't be described in decibels. Rather, you feel like the noise can literally knock you over. Your entire body vibrates. It's a total sensory experience, and for many it is addictive. Some fans travel in motor homes from race to race. Stock cars and the men who drive them are their life. Indeed, they display their loyalties by wearing team hats and jerseys. When meeting someone, it's, "Hello. Are you a Terry Labonte? A Jeff Gordon?" The answer is either affirmative or negative, or "No, I'm a Tony Stewart." They identify themselves by the names of their heroes.

Spiritual Giants Beware!

The old adage says, "There's nothing new under the sun." Hero worship is common throughout history. Christians, of course, eschew the notion of worshipping any mere mortal, but they hold heroes of the faith in high regard. And sometimes they look to a heroic action, office, or status for their source of inspiration. The apostle Paul, who writes 1 Corinthians, chooses not to exalt, but to debunk, three: the great communicator, the spiritual giant, and the martyr.

First of all, it's important to note that Paul uses the first-person singular here. He's not about to level any criticism where he is not the first target. And he's not necessarily referring to types of heroes, but may be simply acknowledging the heroic spiritual fantasies that can influence us as we deal with our egos and our significance in "the body of Christ." His target audience, the Corinthian Church, was very keen to be visible and active in spiritual gifts. In fact, they were so keen they were competing with one another to the point where spiritual capabilities were seen as accomplishments rather than tools for service. It was all about "me," with little regard for "us." So Paul writes an essay beginning with Chapter 12 through to Chapter 14 to dispel their ignorance and to establish "love" as the "highest goal" (14:1) of the truly spiritual person. Chapter 13 is right in the middle, and is without doubt the essential "meat" of the teaching.

The Corinthians had obviously heard about the Day of Pentecost when the Church got its start (Acts 2). They were impressed with *glossolalia* ("tongues"), the ability to speak in unlearned languages under the influence of the Holy Spirit. It doesn't appear they were concerned about the message ("the wonderful things God has done," Acts 2:11b);

they just wanted to be the "messenger." What a thing to be able to command a crowd with your proficiency in the languages of both men and of angels! I don't know about Paul's day, but today there are over 3,000 languages (to say nothing of dialects) spoken. As for the languages in heaven, I've been told by several rabbis (tongues not necessarily in cheek) that there's only one: Hebrew! But here you have someone fluent in all earthly and heavenly languages. How impressive is that?

"Not very," says Paul, "if all you are is a talking head and not a beating heart." If you're all about self-love, you might as well be beating your head on a brass drum. If you're not adding value, you're only adding noise.

That, by the way, is what love does: it adds value. It seeks the highest good for God and neighbor. It has very little, if anything, to do with how we feel. It's an action word. Or, to put it theologically, it's volitional. "Like" is a passive word; it's emotional. This is why it would have been an impossible task if Jesus had told us to "like" our enemies. "Love" is another matter; we can add value to and seek the highest good of someone we dislike. We simply choose to do what's right.

So much for the great communicator. What about the spiritual giant? You know, the person who not only reads your mail but seems to be able to read God's mail as well! Here's someone truly impressive and more than slightly intimidating. They know all of God's secret plans as well as everything about everything. On top of that, they can move mountains at a word of command. This is someone whose future is guaranteed—think book sales, stock-market success, television talk shows, whatever. There's an air of divinity here.

Now, we know Paul is drawing a caricature and is exaggerating for the sake of emphasis. He seems to be veritably hyperventilating with hyperbole. But he does so because of the serious nature of spiritual hubris. Spiritual gianthood is the goal of so many preachers, books, seminars, and movements. It's all about impressing people; it's spiritualized pride. It has nothing to do with serving people. That's why Paul discounts it. Religion is always trumped by relationship. I may be great in my own eyes, and impressive in the eyes of others, but if my gifts serve myself only, I self-marginalize and cast myself on the trash heap of the vain. I think I'm somebody, but really I'm nobody.

The martyr is the tough one. Who is going to speak ill of some-one who impoverishes himself for the poor and/or dies for a great cause? Who is going to find fault with self-sacrifice? Who is going to diminish the memory of the fallen? Who can question the motive? Paul wisely questions his own. He's implying that being right in an argument or in life can be beguiling and compelling enough to die for. It's the ultimate turning on your heel, storming out, and slam-ming the door behind you. You leave your interlocutor's jaw slack with no opportunity of a comeback. You make your point by dying for it. You may be dead wrong, but now you're dead—and no one can do or say anything about it. The less informed onlooker will see only your martyrdom, not your intransigence, and praise you with great praise. Heaven, however, will be silent. It does not recognize self-will.

What Love Is Like

So, not only is love the great theme of heaven, it is also the great theme of a great life. A well-lived life has a well-worn heart. The egotist goes to his grave with his heart well preserved—he gave it to no one. The question is, what is love? Paul gives no answer. But he does tell us what it's like:

> *⁴Love is patient and kind. Love is not jealous or boastful or proud ⁵or rude. It does not demand its own way. It is not irritable, and it keeps no record of being wronged. ⁶It does not rejoice about injustice but rejoices whenever the truth wins out. ⁷Love never gives up, never loses faith, is al-ways hopeful, and endures through every circumstance. (1 Cor. 13:4–7)*

Doesn't it seem that love appears to be everything that human na-ture isn't? I've been jealous, boastful, proud, rude, demanding, irri-table (some would say irritating), and have kept score when I've been wronged. I've also had that little bit of silent satisfaction at a rival's misfortune. Yes, I'm all this and probably much more. But then, so are you. Aren't we all? Little wonder that dysfunction has such long shelf life in human history. Love calls us higher.

It calls us to patience, kindness, truthfulness, determination, faith, hope, and perseverance. Love would see us long-suffering rather than ruthless, gentle rather than harsh, straightforward rather than dissembling, faithful rather than fickle, trusting rather than cynical, strong rather than weak. In a word, love makes us grow up. It eschews childishness and embraces adulthood. The immature, at best, can only receive love. The mature can give it away.

It's human nature to want to be the great communicator, the spiritual giant, the martyr, the hero—and we bring with our striving all the baggage outlined here. This is why churches are sometimes war zones rather than houses of God. Paul stresses that the gifts of the Spirit are temporary tools for the short term. Love is for the long term. Gifts are partial. Love is complete.

> *8Prophecy and speaking in unknown languages and special knowledge will become useless. But love will last forever! 9Now our knowledge is partial and incomplete, and even the gift of prophecy reveals only part of the whole picture! But when understanding comes, these partial things will become useless.*
>
> *11When I was a child, I spoke and thought and reasoned as a child. But when I grew up, I put away childish things. 12Now we see things imperfectly as in a cloudy mirror, but then we will see everything with perfect clarity. *All that I know now is partial and incomplete, but then I will know everything completely, just as God now knows me completely.*
>
> *13Three things will last forever—faith, hope, and love—and the greatest of these is love. (1 Cor. 13:8–13)*

No need for me to rhapsodize here. The words speak eloquently for themselves. Just note the contrast between religion in space and time as partial and incomplete and love as perfect and complete both here and in the heavenlies. Our current knowledge is growing so slowly we appear more stuck than moving. Love is dynamic, not static. Any attempt to project absolutism is a nonstarter because our grasp of heavenly realities is a work in progress. We will one day have perfect knowledge, but not now. In the present the true believer must link arms with the seeker—we're fellow pilgrims more blind than sighted, learning to love a God who first loved us. Just as we loved our earthly parents long before we really knew them, so too we love a heavenly Father we've never seen and hardly know. Our hope is that one day we'll "know as we are known."

In the meantime, love will not have us merely proclaiming and celebrating the gospel. The only way a broken world will see that "God so loved the world" is if "the Church so loves the world." We've got to be more than a voice; we've got to be hands at work.

So let me tell you about two local churches I know well. One is large, the other medium-sized. They are in neighboring African countries and each is in its capital city. Let's call the large one Church A and the other Church B. They represent two different Protestant denominations, and both churches, by the way, were founded about forty years ago by North American missionaries, one American, the other Canadian.

Church B is essentially a meeting place. The people gather, sing some songs, the preacher preaches, then everyone disperses. During the service the children exit for Sunday school. As for the youth, they're in the service, but their main event happens on Saturday afternoons when they gather for an informal Bible study, some sports activity, and some food. The Sunday meeting is high in energy, with lots of noise. The people appear to be genuinely committed to the truth of the gospel, affirming any reference to Jesus, salvation, healing, and deliverance with heartfelt "Amens!" Their singing is beautiful, the preaching is urgent, and the prayers are intense.

Two-thirds of the congregation are made up of women. They sing and pray with a desperate edge. You get the sense that behind the colorful dresses and the beseeching faces is a depth of suffering. Many of them are thin—too thin. But, thinnest of all is the veneer the pastor has spread: "No, Pasta Jim, there's no HIV in our church. We teach against sexual sin." And, if the pastor says there's no HIV, there's no HIV. He's the man of God. What he says is true.

The pastor is the guardian and manager of Church B's subculture. "Holiness" is a core value. He preaches against smoking, drinking, and fornication. There is more than enough evidence of the brokenness resulting from drunkenness and promiscuity to support his thesis.

The women in the congregation know this only too well. Societal evil and family dysfunction are "the wages of sin." In Church B you hide or deny any of the wages that have come to you. And, if you suffer from "the slim disease," you are supported by the pastor and the people who describe your condition as "tuberculosis" or "pneumonia" or "kidney failure" or whatever. Anything but admit your affliction is sexually transmitted. Anything but HIV.

In Church B anyone on the "outside" who wants in is welcome. There is rest and healing offered, but there's no outreach to the outside. When you're in, you're in, free and protected from sin. The world is evil and we Church B people refer to it as "them." As for ourselves, we are "us." We will go to "them" in a programmed outreach kind of way with the objective of bringing them in. But live with them? Mix with them? Stay in the dark place? No, for surely temptation will overtake us. Remember, it's them or it's us. Choose the redeemed.

Frankly, Church B reminds me a lot of me. I've spent most of my life walking by on the other side. I've been self-satisfied and content in being separated from the world, pleased to be in the world, not of it. Comfortable as a pharisee, my voice surely would have been among those condemning Jesus for being a friend of prostitutes and sinners. Yep, I'm a Church B kind of guy.

But things are changing for me. The change started about ten years ago when I accepted the pastorate of a large church in a major city. It was a prosperous upper-middle-income Church B kind of church. A multimillion-dollar structure, it was located in the poorest part of town. It was characterized by a benign and righteous insularity until a young couple joined the staff a few years before my arrival. They started reaching out to the poor, first by living among them, second by establishing a powerful ministry to street kids and the children of single-parent households. The church became central to all of this. To its credit, the church funded this new ministry and even provided volunteers to help. When I came on the scene, I quickly embraced this new dimension; I started to connect with various street ministries in town, and developed, in concert with the young staff couple, a broader relationship with justice-seeking ministries like the Salvation Army. We began to feed and clothe the poor, especially focusing on single-parent homes. There was a distinct domino effect to this; the front rows of our church began to fill with single moms, ex-convicts, substance abusers, homosexuals, and prostitutes. Not everyone was pleased. One prominent member came to me one day and said, "Pastor, we've never had a leader so effective in reaching out to the community." Pause. "But it's not our community." He didn't suggest I stop, but he was certainly in discomfort. Love has a way of forcing us out of our comfort zone.

My church (me included) was on its way from being a Church B to becoming a Church A. As it turned out, my calling to the victims of HIV/AIDS occurred while I was in the midst of this transformation. I eventually resigned from the church so that Kathy and I could focus on the pandemic and its victims full-time. Over the past number of years I've seen a lot of Church B's, both in Africa and in the West, becoming Church A's.

So here's Church A. Yes, it too has meetings with singing, preaching, and praying—all vital elements in any church culture. But the church has something else. Instead of seeing the community in which the churchgoers live as "them" or outsiders, they see "us." Indeed, they see their city and even their nation as "us." To borrow from the creatively named toy store Toys 'R Us, this church could call itself Orphans and Widows 'R Us. Love for neighbor is the fuel that sustains their work.

Reading their weekly bulletin, their monthly letter, or their annual report, your mind boggles at what this African church is doing. They have several community-based development projects. For example: I visited one of forty-three bore holes they had sunk in surrounding rural areas. The fresh water is not only transformative for the people in terms of sanitation, hygiene, and general health, but it has also provided employment and management opportunities for the people; the boreholes are controlled by fences and gates; certain salaried people have keys and the responsibility of providing ingress, access, and security; others have water delivery responsibilities; others maintenance, and so on, all supervised by a community committee. In fact, the national leadership sees this church as expert in development. It has an ever-growing health care ministry employing doctors, nurses, lab technicians, and other trained medical staff who provide health care to thousands of the poor. Vital to this is their HIV/AIDS ministry, which oversees the care of those in various stages of deterioration. This church also administers antiretroviral therapies and is active in famine relief, agricultural projects, infrastructural development for rural communities, child advocacy, literacy education, schools, clinics, and a hospital. Scores of volunteers assist the church's programs, especially in the area of home-based care for the dying. They and the church leaders provide counseling services for people living with HIV/AIDS. Their Sunday services teach about HIV/AIDS; their goal is to mainstream HIV/AIDS into their church culture. They are active in HIV/AIDS prevention programs and educating the public, with a view to reducing the stigma and discrimination associated with the disease. Why, they even have someone, as I write, developing HIV/AIDS texts in Braille for the blind, and signing courses for the deaf.

Little wonder that Church A is large and growing. What can the Almighty do with a church like this but bless it? They are salt and light in a dark place. The nation "sees their good works, and glorifies their father, who is in heaven." They are known as a church with a heart.

Church B continues to "hop and peck," doing church in the traditional way. Church A has seen a new horizon of proactive love, and has become a model for all the world to see. This church is one of the reasons why I believe, in spite of the dark storm of HIV/AIDS blanketing the continent, that one day God will bless the world out of Africa.

If someone lived to be fifty,
they were old...

*I*t was a dismal, dreary, damp morning as I pressed my face against the windowpane. Everything outside was washed in gray. It was a day to snuggle under the covers and sleep in, but I couldn't. I was too excited.

Dad was taking me to a funeral! A country funeral, 40 miles away! This, for a five-year-old boy, had the makings of a huge adventure. Traveling 40 miles of muddy roads held huge promise. We'd probably get stuck and a team of horses would have to pull us out. The car's radiator would probably boil over, requiring a search in ditches and fields for standing water. And Dad would probably pick up some stranded driver and there would be the fun of hearing his story.

Then we might, if I was lucky, run out of gas. This would mean a visit to the nearest farm, running the gamut of farm animals and curious (but not vicious, I hoped) dogs. The farmer's wife would invite us in for tea, and we'd leave an hour or so later with a couple of gallons of "purple gas," which was sold at subsidized prices for farm machinery use only, not for cars—if the police caught you burning purple gas in your car, you got a healthy fine. Wow! Wouldn't it be great if the police stopped us and fined us! Dad would have to explain the situation, tell the cop he was a pastor, the policeman would apologize, he'd fuss over me and maybe show me his gun!

I loved funerals. In town they would start with the local florist bringing long rectangular cardboard boxes full of flowers to our house. Mom was the flower arranger. She'd pull out vases and slowly create funereal bouquets. *The kitchen floor would be covered with clippings, stray baby's breath, remnants of fern, ribbons, and cellophane. There would be a flower smell all through the house, and my brother and I would play with the boxes. Our favorite game was to lie in them and pretend they were caskets. The trick was to lie there totally expressionless and "dead" while the other guy performed the funeral. We'd tire of this, especially if the "preacher" ran out of material, and we'd take the boxes to the top of the stairs and hurl ourselves down in them like sleds on a bumpy hill. Then we'd help Mom carry the floral arrangements over to the church. This was always a tense exercise—not the carrying, but the anticipation that maybe the body had arrived. I had this fearful fascination with looking at the departed. I felt like I was being let in on a dark secret.*

My reverie at the window was cut short by a call from downstairs. "Jimmy!" shouted my father, "Let's go." I ran down the stairs like I was running to the circus. There was nothing like a funeral to make a kid feel truly alive.

When I burst outside, the smell of a wood fire told me the adventure had already begun. Dad had lit a small fire under the car's engine. He often did this in the winter to warm the oil pan in order for the engine in the old '47 Pontiac to turn over and start. He couldn't afford a block heater. Through trial and error over the years, he had developed this risky undertaking into an art form (my mom didn't even want to hear about it). But, this wasn't winter, it was a cold, wet day in early April. His goal this time was to dry out the ignition wires, which had been transplanted from a '36 Chevy. They were spongy and decrepit, totally useless when wet. But, once dried, they performed in a mediocre sort of way, and Dad was able to make his pastoral rounds with only a modicum of hiccoughs and burps from the jury-rigged, rasping engine. The key was to avoid driving through puddles.

It had taken two hours with Dad carefully tending the burning coals, but the car started. Coughing and belching smoke, the old Pontiac came to life and, with one windshield wiper thrashing erratically, we were off.

The first few miles were uneventful. The road leading into our small Saskatchewan town was well graveled and solid. It was when we got to the county line that we saw we had our work cut out for us. The road was a long, straight, ribbon of black mud bounded by what looked like an inland sea. The fields were totally covered with about 6 inches of standing water and we couldn't even see the ditches on either side of the road. Never one to yield to the elements or reason, my dad set his jaw, jammed the old car into second gear, and attacked.

I've often thought that in the history of driving, Saskatchewan drivers in the 1950s must have been some of the best. They knew how to drive on the edge by the seat of their pants. We knew a farmer, Stan Billings, who used to drive his '49 Ford from his farmhouse across the fields to the county road in the depth of winter. At the first snowfall he would create a "track"; that is, his tires would compact the snow, leaving two ribbons of icy white across the field. Then, every day, especially after successive snowfalls, he'd drive over these tracks. Each passage built the tracks up a bit more. By midwinter they were anywhere from 2 to 3 feet high, bounded by unpacked, drifted snow. He would drive that route without slipping off, and do so without the benefit of snow tires. In the spring the surrounding snow would melt long before the compacted tracks. They looked like train rails made out of ice. When we'd remark on his achievement, Stan would shrug and say, "Nah, there's not much to it. You just gotta stay on the tracks." Exactly.

Dad knew that to negotiate a muddy road, you had to keep your momentum. Slip, slide, bump, and splash, but keep going. Don't slow down. If you did, you were like a moving motorboat losing its plane, and you'd sink to your axles. After about 10 miles of teeth-gritting, bone-shaking slip-sliding, we made it to the next county road, which, to our relief, was relatively passable. We did encounter one or two huge puddles on the way. When we hit the first one, Dad uttered an ominous, "Uh, oh," but the Pontiac kept running. "Guess the Vaseline worked," I heard him say to himself. In a stroke of brilliance, he'd coated the ignition wires that morning with Vaseline! Saskatchewan drivers not only knew how to drive, they knew how to improvise.

To my amazement, we made the next 30 miles without incident. We did have to stop a couple of times and dig the "gumbo" (thick, clay-like mud) from the wheel wells. So much had built up that the wheels could hardly turn, but this ritual was par for the course. We didn't run out of gas, the rad didn't boil over, we didn't get stuck. But I had the thrill of my young life when, on a straight, empty stretch of good road, Dad sat me on his lap and let me steer the car! (This was the first of many times I would do so in the future. When I got bigger, I'd sit right beside him and steer. When I was twelve he taught me how to operate the controls. When I was sixteen I passed my driver's test with flying colors.)

As we approached the little country church, it began to rain heavily. Climbing the hill up to the quaint building was a challenge. Dad had to fully employ his driving skills. When we pulled up and parked, I noticed that the cemetery was on the side of the hill next to the church. There was a large pile of freshly dug earth near a weathered wooden cross. "I guess that's where they're gonna bury her," I thought. People were gathering, most of them arriving by horse-drawn wagons. A few had cars. One or two drove trucks. A group of three came on a tractor. Several walked. They were all in their countrified "Sunday-go-to-meetin'" clothes. Everyone was soaking wet.

As Dad went into the church to meet with the bereaved family, there was a break in the weather. I decided to look around. The church building intrigued me; it was made of wood with what had once been white-painted siding. Now the siding was totally gray and weatherbeaten. The top of the steeple had fallen off and was still on its side about 20 feet from the wooden cross. The windows had all been boarded up, although someone had removed the boards from one, revealing plastic sheeting in place of glass. I noticed that the sides of the church seemed to be swollen, as if someone had pumped it up with an air pump. Dad told me later it was because the church had been used for thirty years as a granary. "Nothing tests the structural strength of a building like storing grain in it. Eventually the sides of most buildings swell out and burst. This is why you see so many derelict buildings on farms," he said. When a building withstood this slow torture, it was a well-built structure. Obviously, this beaten-up old church was solid, but today it was full of sorrow. I heard the weeping as I walked over to check out the cemetery.

My mother had taught me to read when I was four. Now, at five, I could read at a Grade Four level. I had no problem reading the grave markers. "Brenden, beloved son of the John and Mary Martin, born 1902, died 1908, 'Suffer the little children.'"

"Myrtle, wife of Allan, mother of Aimee and Mark, born 1920, died 1946, 'Rest in Peace.'" "Chilton, George, 1922–1943." "Anderson, Anne, beloved daughter of Kenneth and Alice, born 1931, died 1949." I could add and subtract as well as read, and I wondered at the number of grave markers standing over so many young people. Life was hard in the early 1900s. I was to learn years later that if someone lived to be over fifty, they were old. Life expectancy was low. War, disease, and hunger took its toll.

I ran back to the church when I heard the singing. In plaintive and slightly off-key tones the assembled congregation were singing "Shall we gather at the river..."; the only "musical" accompaniment was my father's loud, commanding baritone:

> *Shall we gather at the river,*
> *Where bright angel feet have trod,*
> *With its crystal tide forever*
> *Flowing from the throne of God?*

> *(Chorus):*
> *Yes, we'll gather at the river,*
> *The beautiful, the beautiful river,*
> *Gather with the saints at the river*
> *That flows from the throne of God.*

> *Soon we'll reach the shining river,*
> *Soon our pilgrimage will cease;*
> *Soon our happy hearts will quiver*
> *With the melody of peace.*

I looked at these simple country saints with their wet, bedraggled clothing. As they sang, they seemed transported to another country, another realm, another dimension. Their faces shone, and everyone seemed on tiptoe. It was as though their loved one was standing on tiptoe herself, but on the other side, smiling, waving, and beckoning them to join her. I was only five, but I was in awe.

Dad preached a short sermon and then led the pallbearers carrying the plain pine box out to the gravesite. It was raining again, a soft, soaking rain. The little congregation followed, like ducklings following their mother. Everyone stood silently around the grave, the pallbearers on either side. While Dad took a moment to find the appropriate scripture to read, one of the pallbearers shifted, and we heard a distinct splash. I was next to him, looked down into the grave, and saw it had at least 2 feet of water at the bottom. Before I could make eye contact with Dad, it happened.

One side of the grave collapsed, throwing two pallbearers into the water at the bottom, the casket on top of them. There was a flurry of action—slipping, shouting, screaming, crying, words of instruction, grunting, lifting, pushing, and helping—until, finally, the muddy pallbearers were back on terra firma, the casket poised for committal, and Dad—totally unfazed—ready to read the scripture and pray. I was astonished at how quickly we had journeyed from peace to bedlam back to peace again. Everyone retained their dignity, the departed was summarily dispatched, the bereaved were comforted, and Dad and I were back in our car. The entire event had taken an hour. On the way home we got stuck, and spent the night in the car.

A few months ago I stood at the side of a grave in rain-soaked central Zambia. The red earth was a sea of mud. The mourners wept with dignity. They sang with assurance. The grave markers all spoke of good people dying young. It was Saskatchewan all over again. Only this time, the grave didn't collapse.

Chapter 5

"Why Does He Allow a Girl Like Me to Be So Abused?"

I'm sitting with twelve young adults in a twilit room next to the platform of a large church in Lusaka, Zambia. All of them are HIV positive. We're talking about suffering. I'm riveted by what I hear.

"Hello, Pastor, my name is Nicholas. I'm twenty-four years old and I'm finishing my master's degree in engineering. I was orphaned at age twelve and lived on the street. This church found me, fed me, and educated me. They gave me a foster family and I love them as much as I loved my natural parents. One day when I was eighteen, I was crossing the street when a bus hit me. Its brakes had failed. I was thrown right across the intersection and I lay there unconscious and bleeding badly. They tell me it took twenty minutes for a truck to arrive and take me to the hospital. I was almost dead from loss of blood. They gave me five transfusions over the next few days. Unfortunately, some of the blood was tainted with HIV. So, even while I recovered from the accident over the following months, it seemed I was constantly sick—coughs, colds, the flu. Many times they thought I had malaria. But I was always coming down with something.

"We all thought it was because I was weak from the accident. It never occurred to us that it was the transfusions. Two years ago I was skin and bone. I was covered with sores and I had oral thrush. I don't know how I made it to church one Sunday, but that was the day our pastor had himself tested for HIV right there on the platform in front of us all. Until then I had avoided testing. But now, seeing my own pastor tested, I thought maybe I should follow his example, so I did. I was scared, but I did it. I was depressed by the result, but also relieved. At least I knew what my problem was. But, facing a death sentence shakes your soul. 'Why is this happening to me?' I asked. 'What have I done to deserve this?'

"In my confusion and despair I turned to God, the very God who had looked the other way when I stepped in front of that bus, and I cried for help. It was about then that this group of people living with HIV/AIDS was formed in our church. I joined. Found I wasn't alone. Then the church received its first shipment of antiretrovirals. They put us all on the program, and look at us! We're all still HIV positive, but we're healthy. I've gained 70 pounds! And I'm back at the university. The side effects of the ARVs are nasty, but when I want to complain, I consider the alternative. I thank God for this group, this church, and for the Canadians providing us with ARVs."

"Hello, Pastor, my name is Veronica. I just turned twenty-one last week. I'm a widow with three children and I'm HIV positive. I have attended this church all my life. I sing in the choir. In fact, that's where I met my husband—he sang bass. We married when I was seventeen and he was twenty-two. I didn't know he was HIV positive. Neither did he. Last year, on his deathbed, he told me he had had a lot of girlfriends before and during our marriage. He said he slept with more than thirty women a year. I had no idea. I assumed he was faithful to me.

"Somewhere along the line he infected me with HIV. Perhaps it was in our second year when he wanted dry sex. I didn't want it, but what could I do? So I used the powder and the sex hurt and tore me. I suffered quietly, but I began to dread sex. I think I was pretty vulnerable to infection then. Anyway, here I am, a widow, HIV positive, and one of my children, the two-year-old, is also positive. ARVs are keeping us healthy. At least I won't die until the kids are teenagers. That comforts me. And, I'm grateful for a job. I'm a domestic for one of the internationals who attends our church."

"Hello, Pastor, my name is Grace. I'm twenty-two and I graduate this year with a bachelor's degree in education. I was very bright in high school and skipped two grades. I had my bachelor of arts by the time I was nineteen. My parents were very loving to each other and to us kids. My father was a businessman and he was able to pay my university tuition costs. But then, on my twentieth birthday, they were driving from Kitwe back to Lusaka when the trailer behind a truck traveling in the opposite direction came loose and hit their car. It cut through the car like a knife. My parents didn't have a chance. I was devastated. I cried for weeks. And it wasn't just for sorrow. I was angry too. Angry at God. Angry at my father's brothers who took away our house, furniture, and everything they could get their hands on. They did this freely because my parents had left no will. I was out, and had to live with friends. As for university, how could I pay the fees? I had already registered for my first year in education but now I had to go to the registrar and tell him I couldn't pay. He listened to my story and then proposed I pay another way.

"I was desperate, felt I had lost my faith, and was poor, so I did it. I became his girlfriend and attended classes for free, but I felt cheap. I felt like a prostitute. After the first year I broke up with him, and didn't know where to turn. My friend suggested I come to this church and talk to the pastor. Frankly, I was turned off faith, but I needed help. So I came here, the pastor heard my story, and he arranged for a family in the church to take me in, and he organized funds from a donor overseas to pay my university costs. I was thrilled! But shortly afterwards I became ill. It was like a bad case of malaria that wouldn't go away. The pastor suggested I go for testing. I did, and they told me I had HIV. This was the final straw. I'd lost my parents, I'd prostituted myself, and now this? Where was the justice? Where was God? Why me? I'm still angry and I'm not sure I should even be in this group, but I need the ARVs. ..."

A Theology of Suffering

The rest of the group told their stories as well. They ran the gamut from rape to intravenous drug use to commercial sex to casual sex. Each one had incurred serious loss, had endured years of suffering, and had wrestled with disappointment with God. All but one were in their twenties and were mature beyond their years. Suffering will do that.

Cyril, the twenty-eight-year-old Chinese-Zambian, who had contracted HIV through sleeping around, looked at me with pools of hurt in his eyes and said, "Talk to us, Pastor. Talk to us about what the Bible says about suffering."

"What have I got to say to you?" I responded. "When it comes to suffering, you are the veterans. I'm the junior player."

"No, no, that's not what I mean, "Cyril said. "What I mean is give us the theology of suffering. We need to find some meaning in all of this. You're the pastor. You tell us. Are we suffering for nothing?"

"Well, first of all," I began, "I'm way over my head here. Your stories have touched me deeply and I feel blessed by your sharing them with me and very challenged by the depth of your life experiences. I feel shallow by comparison. In fact, due to my limited experience with suffering, I've had to rely on people like you, authors,* and a lot of biblical study to have anything worthwhile to say. But you've asked, so here goes.

"Let me start with a story. One morning in Jerusalem my wife Kathy bathed the cat. Cats, as you know, hate water. The very moment Kathy headed for the tub, cat under her arm, there was a sudden demonstration of splayed claws, fur on end, and unearthly snarls. During the bath itself, it sounded as if every stray cat in the neighborhood was protesting nuclear warfare in unison. When it was over, with her wet fur, she looked gaunt and greasy, and she had terror in her eyes. It took twenty minutes for her claws to retract. As she began an hour of preening her violated fur, Kathy, whose arms were badly scratched, said to me, 'It'll be days before she trusts me again.' The cat's hour of suffering meant a week without purring.

---

* See Carl Michaelson, *Faith for Personal Crises*; Leslie D. Weatherhead, *Salute to a Sufferer*; George A. Buttrick, *God, Pain, and Evil*; C.S. Lewis, *The Problem of Pain*.

"The bath was for the cat's good, but she didn't know it, resented it deeply, felt violated, and went into a week-long sulk. In fact, if her god had not been her belly, and her belly didn't strongly identify our home with food, I wouldn't have been surprised if she had left home for good and joined the garbage cat fellowship. The food there may not have been as succulent, but at least you wouldn't have to suffer the indignities of cleanliness!"

"Israelis have cats for pets?" Jeremiah blurted, astonished.

"Not just Israelis. Canadians. Americans. Europeans. Much of the world keep cats as pets," I answered.

"In my village we eat them," muttered Amos. "At least we did until there were no more."

After the laughter had died down, I continued. "Now, we know every analogy fails somewhere. I'm not suggesting we're cats, but there are some parallels between my story and what we go through when we suffer.

"Before I talk about the 'Big Questions' in suffering, let me make two foundational statements. First of all, suffering is less a physical challenge and more a spiritual challenge. Second, no suffering we undergo as God's children will defeat God's purpose for our lives; he will always use it for good, whether it's for us, our world, for himself, or all of the above. There are no surprises for God because he is omniscient. There are no forces able to thwart his plan, for he is omnipotent. When God is in the mix, there is meaning. Always.

"All of us have had a friendly wrestling match at some time or other in our lives, usually as children. Perhaps, if you're a parent, you've wrestled with your kids. Sometimes, as happened to Kathy and our daughter, Katie, several years ago, somebody gets hurt. In this instance they bumped heads, enough to raise respective 'goose eggs' with more than a howl or two of pain. But there were no tears even though Katie was only five. Why? Because immediately after the skull-to-skull collision, Katie looked into her mother's eyes. I guarantee that if she had seen anger, displeasure, or disapproval she would have cried. But she saw playfulness—rattled cranium playfulness, mind you—but playfulness nonetheless. Somehow the surprise and silliness of cracked heads neutralized the pain. With much laughter they rubbed each other's foreheads and carried on. Suffering is less a bump on the head and more a look in the eye.

"Physical pain is not the ultimate concern. Indeed there are those who argue that pain is the small question in suffering. The bigger question is 'Why has this happened?' The biggest, 'Why has this happened to me?' is the killer. That question, if left unanswered, can destroy faith, relationships, and life itself.

"'Why has this happened to me?' has a companion: 'Why didn't this happen to John?' It's a kind of subtle covetousness. We envy John's freedom from suffering but, in a perverse sort of way, think that he would have been a much more suitable candidate for pain. One thing is clear: we don't deserve this. It's unjust. Unfair."

"Just a minute, Pastor," Grace says. "I didn't think that way. I don't think that way. I'm happy that others are HIV-free."

"Okay. But tell me, Grace. Have you ever looked at some young woman at university, living a wild life, carefree, and seemingly immune from trouble? Have you ever felt that it's unfair that her irresponsible life should be rewarded?"

"Maybe. Maybe once or twice, but I didn't dwell on it."

"Good for you. But the point is we do look at others and compare ourselves to them. We see the contrast and sometimes we envy, sometimes we gloat. It's tough to be neutral, especially when the other guy seems to be getting a better deal out of life. But here's the point I'm trying to make. We humans are rather weird ducks as contrasted to the rest of creation. Animals ask only for food, shelter, and sex. We ask for meaning. To ask 'Why me?' is to express belief in some kind of ultimate plan. We value rhyme and reason. We seek 'a better country.' Our hearts tell us intuitively that the 'far country' exists, and its maker exists. So we look beyond when we ask 'Why me?' We want to know if our suffering is seen, heard, or felt in heaven. If it is, how does it factor into the will of our Creator?"

Grace again. "In one of my psychology classes we talked about suffering and the professor reminded us that Freud said that much of our suffering is self-inflicted. It's our way of escaping responsibility for our actions. Frankly, I was offended. How could my suffering at the death of my parents be self-inflicted? And how could my HIV be self-inflicted?" Pausing a moment she thought about what she had just said. Before someone else could point it out, she admitted, "Well, I suppose I did choose to sleep with the registrar, but only in order to go to school. But I certainly would not have done so if I'd known his HIV status."

"I think the point Freud was making," I answered, "was expressed well by an author I read who said suffering can be 'an opiate against pain,' our 'recoil from an active mastery of life.' Yet another suggested that we accuse ourselves with diseases to pre-empt the accusation of others. You don't hit someone when they're down. Knowing this we will sometimes find ourselves ill to avoid the judgment of others. It's a similar mechanism to putting yourself down before someone else does. I've had doctors tell me that they have patients who have no physical reason for illness, but they're ill all the same. The doctors see it as a control mechanism. When you're sick, you can get your own way, receive sympathy, get attention, and totally avoid responsibility. Illness can be the great friend of the passive noncombatant in the battle of life. And, to be brutal, we can sometimes use suffering aggressively: 'If you hadn't been so mean to me, this never would have happened.'"

"But Freud lived in an HIV-free world," said Nicholas. "We've been blind-sided by this thing. We need fresh thinking."

"Maybe," I said, "but before we make an attempt, let me say this. Grace brought up the psychiatrist Freud. Let me bring up two others most of you have studied—the philosopher Nietzsche, and the theologian Kierkegaard. It's been a long time since I read either of these men, but I do remember that both built a fairly positive case for suffering. Nietzsche said that great goals are achieved only through suffering. And Kierkegaard, as you would expect, refers to the Bible, where the apostle Paul said, "Suffering produces endurance, and endurance produces character, and character produces hope" (Rom. 5:3, 4). Kierkegaard saw suffering as instrumental to great achievement. In his view, suffering is not incidental to the process of life; it is the process. Another theologian, John Calvin, saw suffering as a sacrament through which Christians are led 'by the discipline of the cross into deeper knowledge of themselves.' But, I dare say all of these answers must seem a bit thin for someone who's just tested positive for HIV."

"That's for sure," said Veronica. "But, Pastor, I'm not sure Nicholas is right when he says we need new thinking about suffering because of HIV. I think anyone who suffers, suffers. It doesn't matter if it's HIV, cancer, or the loss of a child. Does the Bible say anything about where suffering comes from?"

"Satan!" blurted Cyril. "He's the enemy of our souls. He seeks, kills, and destroys. He's happy to make us suffer."

"That's only partially true," said Reuben, who had been silent until now. He was a Bible college student in his third year of studies. "The Bible says there are a lot of sources for suffering."

"Yeah? Like what?" Cyril asked.

"Well, like disobedience, laziness, foolishness, greed, unfaithfulness, a bad attitude, stuff like that."

"Which are all negative causes," I said. "There are positive sources of suffering as well."

"For instance?" prompted Nicholas.

"We often suffer because we love. The apostle Paul wrote to the Corinthians, 'out of great distress and anguish of heart and with many tears, not to grieve [them] but to let [them] know the depth of [his] love for [them].' You can read about it in 1 Corinthians 2. Like a parent he had deep concern for his 'children.' That kind of concern can produce a lot of suffering. Or, take empathy. The scripture says we're to 'rejoice with those who rejoice; mourn with those who mourn.' We suffer because a brother or sister suffers."

"Where's that?" asked Veronica.

"Romans 12:15."

"Even God suffers because of love," said Reuben. "Back in Genesis, Chapter 6, I think, it says God was so grieved about mankind's behavior his heart 'was filled with pain.' He was distressed when Israel was distressed, and he loved the world so much he sacrificed his only son to save us. I mean, how much did it hurt God the Father to see his 'only begotten son' beaten and crucified?"

"You're sounding like a preacher already," I chuckled.

"Sorry, but I'm really into this subject. Just last month at college we were studying Dietrich Bonhoeffer's book, *The Cost of Discipleship*. We got into a huge discussion about the suffering required of a committed follower of Jesus. I even wrote a paper on it."

"Oh no! Here we go. Another sermon," muttered Veronica, with a smile on her face.

"Go ahead," I said, "give us a quick summary."

A touch reluctant, but eager at the same time, Reuben proceeded. "Maybe the bluntest reference is in Hebrews 11:36–38. It's talking about people who chose to follow the road less traveled—you know, God's way. It says, 'Some faced jeers and flogging, while still others were chained and put in prison. They were stoned; they were sawed in two; they were put to death by the sword. They went about in sheepskins and goatskins, destitute, persecuted and mistreated...' I mean, some of these guys—take Abraham for instance—were very wealthy. They could have lived in luxury, taken it easy, but instead, they chose to pursue a vision of the coming world that saw them rejected by society and marginalized, even by their own families. They suffered, some would say needlessly, but they would say meaningfully, because of the impress of heaven on their hearts and minds."

"Impress. Wow! Big word!" Grace mocked.

"It means stamp, mark."

"I know, I know."

"And there's a lot of other discipleship suffering in scripture. We suffer for Christ's sake, for righteousness' sake, for the Kingdom of God, for the gospel, for resisting Satan, just for being a Christian, for the 'Name,' or even as a test of our integrity. Usually embracing faith is not a way out of problems, it's a way into them."

"So why bother?" Grace whispered, a look of dismissal on her face.

"Because faith is not about now as much as it is about then," I countered. "We're only pilgrims. God has made us for the 'far country.' And it's of such value that he'll even hurt us to keep us on track."

"What? You mean God will cause us to suffer?"

"Well, yes and no. No, he doesn't cause it, but he will allow it. Let me give you an example. When my kids were young, I taught all three how to ride a bicycle. Our oldest, Todd, fell the first time I let go of the seat as I ran beside him, cut his lip, ran into the house for comfort from Kathy, got back on the bike, and rode away. He's been riding ever since. In fact, he rode a motorcycle to university for four years. Jess, our second son, got on the bike and rode like he'd always known how.

Kate, our youngest, well, not only did she fall, but she kept careening into parked cars and stone walls!

"Now, I didn't intend for any of them to fall, but I knew they would, and allowed them to fall. And two out of three did. God allows suffering, I think, because he wants us to learn. He wants us to substitute knowledge for ignorance, wisdom for foolishness, holiness for sin. These processes can't be imposed; they've got to be learned—usually the hard way. But God will not allow something that will defeat his purpose. I didn't allow my children to practise their bike riding in highway traffic. I limited the 'suffering field' because I wanted them to live, not die. And I made sure not to ride the bike for them, which is a huge temptation. We're all fixers, we all want instant solutions, ready and easy answers, one of which is divine healing. We figure the answer to HIV/AIDS is a blitz of healing crusades.

"A young man came to me after I spoke recently at a conference in Seattle, Washington. With a condescending air he told me that my call to the Church to seek justice and minister to orphans and widows was the easy way out.

"'Well, you're just protecting and feeding them. How about healing them?' he said.

"Healing them?

"'Yeah. You know. Signs and wonders. The power of the Spirit, the supernatural.'

"Why should God heal them and not us?" I asked.

"'What? What do you mean?'

"Well, we're all terminal. It's just that HIV/AIDS victims have an accelerated death sentence, complicated by ongoing suffering. I'm going to die, and so are you. Maybe our deaths will include prolonged bouts of suffering too. Or maybe we'll be struck by a car when we walk out of here. But why am I failing them if I don't heal them?

"'Jesus healed the sick,' he challenged.

"Did he heal all of the sick he saw? I lived in Jerusalem for seven years. I'm sure a lot of it today is like it was yesterday. There are scores of halt, lame, and blind in the gates of the Holy City. Lots of pathetic beggars, sad-looking widows, and grubby children. It's my guess that Jesus healed one in 1,000 and only when he was moved by compassion. Most of the time he just tried to be a presence with the broken. His love gave the sufferer dignity and hope.

"My zealous friend slunk away, not at all convinced of what I had said. But suffering is like fire. It purifies us. In 1 Corinthians 3:12–15, it says, 'If any man builds on this foundation [Jesus Christ] using gold, silver, costly stones, wood, hay or straw, his work will be shown for what it is, because the Day will bring it to light. It will be revealed with fire, and the fire will test the quality of each man's work. If what he has built survives, he will receive his reward. If it is burned up, he will suffer loss. …'

"Everything but gold is destroyed by fire. In allowing suffering, God shows us how he cares for us. I mean, he could fix us, heal us, and ignore our character development. He could opt for merely making us happy. Rather, he wants to make us good.

"I'm told that a gold refiner uses fire until he can see his own image in the molten metal. God does the same, using fire he didn't make, fueled by our own ignorance, foolishness, and sin, allowing us to suffer until he can see his own image in us."

"Well, he's certainly allowing a lot of suffering in Africa," said Nicholas. "It's not a fire, it's a holocaust."

"That's why the Church must be proactive and loving in the midst of these sorrows," I said. "The silver lining in the dark cloud of HIV/AIDS is that churches all over the continent are waking up to the needs of the afflicted like never before. They're working cross-denominationally as never before. The true, loving heart of the Church is being revealed, and the noble character of Africa is emerging. I believe God can almost see his face in Africa's gold. And I believe it's only a matter of time, and God will bless the world out of Africa."

"Pastor, please. You must come back to earth," said Grace. "I don't think God has anything at all to do with our suffering. I think it's just bad luck."

"I don't think so. If it's simply a matter of luck, then anything can happen. With God, anything cannot happen. Let me illustrate. Long before Kathy and I taught our children to ride bicycles, we taught them how to walk. To do this we had to let them stumble and fall, sometimes with great fright and tears. But we made sure the stairs were well guarded. We made sure there was no broken glass on the floor, no toxic cleaning fluids, or other unnecessary dangers within the falling area. In other words, we guarded and in a sense prepared the falling area. That way nothing could happen with which our children could not cope. Some distressing things might happen, but it's not true to say anything could happen. Nothing could possibly happen in the falling area from which progress could not be gained. In the same way God knows that nothing can happen in this falling area we call Earth that can of itself destroy his plan and purpose for our lives. He's in charge."

At this point Samara spoke up. Just seventeen, she was the youngest in the group; indeed, this was her first time attending. She had come to the meeting from a women's shelter run by the church. Her face was still swollen and bruised from the beating she had received five nights ago.

Two days before that she had run away from home. She had been caring for her AIDS-stricken mother for two years, and for two years had suffered her dead father's brother's sexual advances. But this time he had arrived drunker than usual and had brutally raped her. With no one to defend her, she ran away, hoping it would be safer on the streets than at home. But her third night on the street proved otherwise. She was dragged by the hair into a dark alley by two teenaged boys, beaten, raped, and left for dead. One of the church's street workers had found her an hour later, had taken her to the hospital, and then to the shelter. She sat before us, broken, silent, an open wound.

"I don't think I believe in God," she whispered. "How can I?" she wept. Tears framed her swollen face, her voice gained strength, and she asked, "If God exists, and he's loving and powerful, then why does he allow suffering? Why does he allow a girl like me to be so abused?" And she buried her tortured face in her scraped, scabbed hands.

I couldn't speak. None of us could. Grace and Veronica went over to her and held her as she sobbed. Their embrace released a deeper level of sorrow, and she began to wail. We were listening to the cry of a broken heart. It eclipsed our reasonable discussion. It scored our hearts like a cat's claws rip our skin. I found myself weeping in my chair.

As Samara's sobbing subsided, we all became quiet, everyone looking troubled, everyone's face tear-streaked. I remember thinking in red-eyed peace after the storm that the question was not 'Why does God allow suffering and evil?', but 'Why do we allow it?' Why do we rape, pillage, and steal? Why do we walk by on the other side when we see the broken? Why do we hoard our goods when most of the world is dying from want? Hold Samara, girls, hold her. Dear God! Let us all hold her. Let the Church hold her. The only thing we can give her is love.**

I returned to my hotel room, emotionally wrung out and troubled. I'd always feared being trite when responding to questions about suffering. Tonight, especially in light of Samara's anguish, was I superficial? Trite? Philosophical? Unreal? Yes, I thought, I was. With a desperation fueled by Samara's grief, I studied long into the night. I read several passages from the Bible, but one passage stood out: Romans 8:12–39.

> [12]So, dear brothers and sisters, you have no obligation whatsoever to do what your sinful nature urges you to do. [13]For if you keep on following it, you will perish. But if through the power of the Holy Spirit you turn from it and its evil deeds, you will live. [14]For all who are led by the Spirit of God are children of God.
>
> [15]So you should not be like cowering, fearful slaves. You should behave instead like God's very own children, adopted into his family—calling him Father, dear Father."* [16]For his Holy Spirit speaks to us deep in our hearts and tells us that we are God's children. [17]And since we are his children, we will share his treasures—for everything God gives to his Son, Christ, is ours, too. But if we are to share his glory, we must also share his suffering. (8:12–17)

"O Samara," I thought, "if only your uncle and those two boys had known they were dead even while they lived. Their sinful nature dictated rape. It ruled them, but only because they let it do so. Had it occurred to them that they didn't have to let sex and violence order their lives? Perhaps they felt victimized by their urges. They were too powerful.

** Author's note: I used fictional names to protect the privacy of those who told their stories to me.

Why didn't some Christian somewhere tell them that if they put their trust in God, his Spirit would powerfully kill their sinful natures and give them freedom and new life? Perhaps they felt like, or maybe even were, orphans, alone and without support or protection. Why didn't a Christian tell them that by allowing their heavenly Father rather than their base desires to lead them, they would receive a new heart, a new spirit, a new view of the world, where slavery to lust would give way to freedom to love?"

This passage sees us putting to death our sinful nature, which has parented us, and being adopted by a new father, one we call Abba (which is Hebrew for "Daddy"). It assures us, even those of us who have only known degradation and despair, that we are being placed in a position of dignity as the adopted children of God. As such, we are to inherit with our Father all the blessedness of his presence, his power, splendor, and perfection—in other words, his "glory." In the manifested explosion of his love, we will "run and not be weary, walk and not faint." We will be loved, cared for, and nurtured forever. With one caveat.

We've got to share in and share with Christ's suffering. We share in it by confessing him as our Savior. His death becomes our death to sin. Through that death we satisfy the punitive demands of a justice rooted in the "apartness," the holiness of God. We share with it by enduring the rejection of men and accepting the sorrow and grief that accrue to someone who insists there's a new world awaiting over the horizon. Society hides its face from someone who, like Christ, dismisses material values and prioritizes servanthood. And, throughout history, Christ's followers have sometimes themselves suffered horrible deaths, just because they believed.

What about HIV? Did Christ suffer from AIDS? No. But like a leper, he was hated, despised, and marginalized. He knew all about stigma and discrimination. We suffer with him in that sense. I think Veronica was right—anyone afflicted with suffering, regardless of the source, suffers. Suffering is suffering. There are no special categories. It's just that HIV has unleashed widespread suffering in our world, the likes of which humankind has never seen before. Suffering is more in our face than it has ever been. God's children are hurting, and the Church has got to hold them, otherwise they're orphaned and alone.

I read on. Still emotionally reeling from the stories I had just heard, the scriptures astonished me with their relevance:

> [35]*Can anything ever separate us from Christ's love? Does it mean he no longer loves us if we have trouble or calamity, or are persecuted, or are hungry, or cold or in danger or threatened with death?...*
> [38]*And I am convinced that nothing can ever separate us from his love. Death can't, and life can't. The angels can't, and the demons can't. Our fears for today, our worries about tomorrow, and even the powers of hell can't keep God's love away.* [39]*Whether we are high above the sky or in the deepest ocean, nothing in all creation will ever be able to separate us from the love of God that is revealed in Christ Jesus our Lord.* (Rom. 8:35, 38–39)

God's word is declaring to Nicholas and Cyril, Veronica and Grace, and all others who are suffering, whether it be because of HIV or some other affliction: "Lose your separation anxiety, your fear of rejection, your sense of abandonment—your suffering has not torn you from God, it has brought you to him. Open your eyes. Look and see whom and what he has placed in your path to care for and comfort you. There is nothing in all creation that has anything to say to or to do with your security. He has made a pact with you. Absolutely everything is irrelevant except his love. He loves you. Period. Rest in that assurance. Your story isn't done. The last chapter will gloriously become the first chapter in an everlasting book with endless pages and inexhaustible delight."

A few years ago I stood in my pulpit in Jerusalem and preached on suffering. I found it difficult. Why? Difficult material? Partly. Unpopular approach to the subject? Maybe. My unfamiliarity with suffering? For sure. But more than all this was my discomfort at seeing Don Browning in the audience. Don, a former seminary classmate of mine, was pastor of one of the toughest parishes in Canada, a maximum-security prison in Edmonton. He preached and lived the gospel every day surrounded by murderers, rapists, and gangsters. Husky and handsome, he was forty-one years old, with a wife and three teenaged children. And, he had two months to live. My friend, Don Browning, had inoperable cancer.

After the sermon he stood with about seven others for prayer, knowing more about suffering than most of us put together. Later, in a conversation over coffee with Kathy and me, he said, "You know what I've learned from this sickness? We're all terminal." He told us of his wife's suffering and anger. Just before he came to Israel, she expressed her suffering in an exasperated outburst: "Why aren't you taking this cancer more seriously? Why aren't you preparing for your death?" Don didn't answer at the time, but as he traveled around Israel, an answer came. His response to her and to us: "Why aren't you preparing for *your* death?"

This stunning question begs another, especially when we ask "Why is this happening to me?" That other question is "Why not? Why not me? Why not you?" We are fellow sufferers. Isn't it about time we joined hands?

Bless the God of Africa

BLESS THE GOD OF AFRICA

1. *Oh see the mighty lion!*
   Head high, the walk of kings,
   His vision keen, his mane aglow,
   Resounding roar, he sings—

(Chorus)

   Africa the glorious!
   Africa the true!
   Africa victorious!
   God grant His grace to you.

2. *Majestic hills, resplendent*
   Vast plains horizons clear,
   Deep rivers flow, huge waters fall,
   In thunders loud we hear

(Chorus)

3. *Her people proud and loving,*
   Strong, lifting up the Name,
   The nations' hope, her Champion
   The Lion, Lamb that's slain

(Chorus)

4. Our spirit is undaunted
   Our love for God undimmed
   His light shines forth, this continent
   With praises shall ascend

(Chorus)

5. Bless the God of Africa!
   Bless our greatest Friend!
   He reigns! We live! We flourish!
   Our worship never ends!

(Chorus)

6. Amen! The orphans answer.
   Amen! The widows cry.
   Amen! The people lift their voice,
   God gives us liberty!

(J. Cantelon, copyright CCG Inc. all rights reserved)

Chapter 6
"Summon Your Might, O God, Show Me Your Strength"

Goodbye, "Gentle Jesus meek and mild." Hello, angry God who shatters heads. Tenderness and terror, affirmation and vilification, compassion and damnation—welcome the bipolar deity who acts with impunity. Or, so it seems when you read the "Titan" that is Psalm 68.

It is called a "song," but it confounds the experts because of its incoherence. It seems to lack structure, flow, design. If anything it appears to be a medley compiled, if not plagiarized, by some junior musician. And yet it has more than a ring of truth to it. It has a visceral, almost primordial appeal. The intuitive knowledge of God, which we all possess, seems to stand up in awe and respect, even as God "arises." It is a song that sticks in the throat, but captivates the mind and uplifts the soul. And, perhaps more than many other psalms, it tells us what motivates the Almighty as he stoops to act in space and time.

The "stickiness" of the lyrics, for the modern reader, consists in the unabashed bashing of enemies' heads (v. 21), and the apparent juvenile joy of the "righteous" at the prospect. God, the terrifying adversary, is cheered on by a bloodthirsty mob eager "to plunge [their] feet in the blood of [their] foes" (v. 23a). Why, they'll even release their dogs to lap up their share (v. 23b)! Call it colorful Middle Eastern hyperbole if you will, but be assured that if ever this psalm is read in a church today, these violent descriptions are often omitted. We prefer to see the wrath of God as a concept. The reality is over the top.

When God Stands Up

This "arising" God is a fascinating idea in scripture. The Hebrew word *qum* (pronounced "coom") simply means "to stand, rise, arise" and is used in modern Hebrew every day in Israel. Yet, in Old Testament usage, it has a number of applications.

It can, of course, simply refer to getting up from a prostrate, kneeling, or sitting position. Or, it can be a preparatory action pursuant to some other action. One of those actions can be showing respect. For example, God commands his people to "rise up" before the elderly: "Rise in the presence of the aged, show respect for the elderly and revere your God. I am the Lord" (Lev. 19:32).

Another example: When Moses entered the "tent of meeting" with the "pillar of cloud" over the entrance, everyone "rose up" at the door of his own tent and worshipped: "Whenever the people saw the pillar of cloud standing at the entrance to the tent, they all stood and worshipped, each at the entrance to his tent" (Ex. 32:10).

"Arising" can also apply to the assumption of leadership. Moses, for instance, "rose" to prophetic status: "Since then, no prophet has risen in Israel like Moses, whom the Lord knew face to face..." (Dt. 34:10). An obscure man by the name of Tola "rose" to become a judge of Israel: "After the time of Abimelech a man of Issachar, Tola son of Puah, the son of Dodo, rose to save Israel" (Judg. 10:1). So, if you're "upwardly mobile" in Israel, you "arise."

Then there is the legal usage of "arise" in the sense that it applies to the "establishment" of a "word" or "witness" or "agreement." It has an especially powerful application relative to the "covenant" between God and his people: "I establish my covenant with you: never again will all life be cut off by the waters of a flood; never again will there be a flood to destroy the earth" (Gen. 9:11).

"Then God said, 'Yes, but your wife Sarah will bear you a son, and you will call him Isaac. I will establish my covenant with him as an everlasting covenant for his descendants after him.'" (Gen. 17:19)

"So Ephron's field in Machpelah near Mamre ... was deeded [yes, "deeded" is *yaqum* in Hebrew] to Abraham as his property in the presence of all the Hittites who had come to the gate of the city. ... So the field and the cave in it were deeded to Abraham by the Hittites as a burial site" (Gen. 23:17–19).

I mentioned a few paragraphs back that "arise" can be applied to "preparatory action pursuant to some other action." Often, that "action" occurs in a martial context. For example, look at Moses, Joshua, and Gideon: "Now a priest of Midian had seven daughters, and they came to draw water and fill the troughs to water their father's flock. Some shepherds came along and drove them away, but Moses got up and came to their rescue and watered the flock" (Ex. 2:16, 17). "Now Joshua sent men from Jericho to Ai, which is near Beth Aven to the east of Bethel, and told them 'Go up and spy out the region'" (Josh. 7:2). "When Gideon heard the dream and its interpretation, he worshipped God. He returned to the camp of Israel and called out, 'Get up! The Lord has given the Midianite camp into your hands'" (Judg. 7:15).

By the way, whether it's Moses, Joshua, Gideon, or some other person moved by the Spirit of God to "arise," the assumption is that God "arises" with them. And, when God "arises" to engage in combat, victory is certain. When God stands up, his enemies go down. But they don't go down easily—they "scatter." The first time this arising–scattering scenario is recorded, Moses is praying before the ark is sent out: "Rise up, O Lord! May your enemies be scattered; may your foes flee before you" (Num. 10:35). Isaiah says, "At the thunder of your voice the peoples flee; when you rise up, the nations scatter" (33:3).

Scattered Enemies

Then there are several references where "scattering" is predicated on a presumed "arising": "He shot his arrows and scattered the enemies" (Ps. 18:14); "with your strong arm you scattered your enemies" (Ps. 89:10b); "all evil doers will be scattered" (Ps. 92:9c). The imagery comes to mind of an anthill that has suddenly been kicked apart, or a hornets' nest that has been knocked down. A frenzied confusion ensues with every "ant" for himself. As for the hornets, they become yellow-jacketed bullets, crazed and angry, looking to kill before they die. Fear, anger, lashing out, transform a retreat into a "scatter."

There are other applications of "scatter" in scripture. The Hebrew word is *putz* (pronounced "pootz") and we see it first in reference to the tower of Babel: "Then they said, 'Come, let us build ourselves a city, with a tower that reaches to the heavens, so that we may make a name for ourselves and not be scattered over the face of the whole earth'" (Gen. 11:4). Ironically, the very thing they feared came upon them, for "the Lord scattered them from there over all the earth" (v. 8). It appears that God has an aversion to hubris.

Some of the references to scattering include armies, sheep, and the nation of Israel. Take a look at these: "The next day Saul separated his men into three divisions; during the last watch of the night they broke into the camp of the Ammonites and slaughtered them until the heat of the day. Those who survived were scattered, so that no two of them were left together" (1 Sam. 11:11), "but the Babylonian army pursued the king and overtook him in the plains of Jericho. All his soldiers were separated from him and scattered, and he was captured" (2 Kings 25:5); "'Woe to the shepherds who are destroying and scattering the sheep of my pasture!' declares the Lord" (Jer. 23:1). "So they were scattered because there was no shepherd, and when they were scattered they became food for all the wild animals" (Ezek. 34:5). "Then Micaiah answered, 'I saw all Israel scattered on the hills like sheep without a shepherd...'" (1 Kings 22:17). Directly or indirectly, the general view in scripture is that all this mayhem is divinely initiated. It is God who scatters.

The Dark Side

And it is also God who shatters—heads, that is. The story of Sisera and Jael comes to mind. In Judges 4 we read about the event; in Chapter 5 we read Deborah's song about it. It's the stuff movies are made of.

You need to read this story for yourself. The climax occurs when Jael kills the Canaanite military commander Sisera by driving a tent peg through his head with a hammer. The narrative in Chapter 4 says she did this while Sisera slept. Deborah's song in Chapter 5 describes her as smashing Sisera's head with a hammer, then driving the peg through his shattered head. Regardless of the chronology of events, Deborah prophetically stated in Chapter 4, "the Lord will hand Sisera over to a woman." God ordained the shattering. Indeed, he was behind it.

The Hebrew word used in this account is *machatz* (pronounced "mahaatz"). It means "to strike, wound severely" and the noun is "severe wound." The blow described by *machatz* is usually devastating and decisive. People struck in this manner usually don't walk away.

The point I'm trying to make here is that in this day of the "seeker-sensitive" and "user-friendly" church, the average congregation is usually in the dark about this "dark side" of God's dealings with humankind. You don't win friends and influence people with words like "annihilate," "shatter," "smite," "crush." Yet, the scriptures use these words to describe God's action again and again. "The Lord is at your right hand; he will crush [*machatz*] kings on the day of his wrath. He will judge the nations, heaping up the dead and crushing [*machatz*] the rulers of the whole earth" (Ps. 110:5–6). "See now that I myself am He! There is no God besides me. I put to death and I bring to life, I have wounded [*machatz*] and I will heal, and no one can deliver out of my hand" (Deut. 32:39). "For he wounds, but he also binds up; he injures [*machatz*], but his hands also heal" (Job 5:18).

But the most vivid passage of all comes from the "Titan" itself: "Surely God will crush [*machatz*] the heads of his enemies, the hairy crowns of those who go on in their sins. The Lord says, 'I will bring them from Bashan; I will bring them from the depths of the sea, that you may plunge your feet in the blood of your foes, while the tongues of your dogs have their share!'" (Ps. 68:21–23). How "in your face" is this? It sounds like the threats of modern-day terrorists. The Almighty seems very angry indeed.

That's why I've got to digress from this psalm for a bit. With more than a small measure of reluctance I'm going to briefly visit the dark side. (Just what you wanted—several pages on the wrath of God, but we've got to cover this. If we're going to understand the significance of righteousness and justice [in Chapter 1], we've got to examine the context making these qualities so vital, so bear with me. We'll get through. Remember, the endgame is the well-being of orphans and widows.)

The Angry God

First of all, wrath is most times, but not always, equivalent to anger. As I read the Old Testament, I often see anger as the stimulus, and wrath as the follow-through: anger, reactive; wrath, proactive. Anger is usually accompanied by strong emotion; wrath is often cool and calculating, but it also can be blindingly devastating. Generally, however, the two go together. Anger is the fuel; wrath, the fire.

Recently, in the vast Serengeti of Tanzania, my wife and I found ourselves caught in the midst of 160 migrating elephants. When we first approached them, the mothers gave some sort of unseen signal and all the little ones clustered in the middle of a mobile guard of maternal menace. Some of the non-nursing mothers took over the point and the rearguard. One of them stopped no more than 10 feet away from our Land Rover, flared her ears, gave a mighty snort, and charged. Bringing her charge up at the last moment, she wheeled away, snorting and stamping. Wisely, we backed off. We knew we were in for trouble if we stayed. The snorting said it all.

In biblical Hebrew, the root from which we derive the verb "to be angry" (*anaph*) means "to snort." The noun (*aph*), used today in modern Hebrew, means "nose." And the nose for ancient Hebrews was the seat of anger. Closely associated with this snort is heat (*hema*)—the heat of a burning fire. King David speaks of the smoke rising from the nostrils of an angry god with "consuming fire" and "burning coals" blazing "from his mouth" (Ps. 18:8). Time and again, "the burning anger" of God is spoken of by the Old Testament writers to the point where a modern reader, perhaps drawn to faith by the appeal of a persuasive preacher, finds himself surprised, repulsed, and afraid of this God who heretofore was a grandfather—certainly not an avenging angel.

Indeed, the Almighty in the Old Testament is downright intimidating. His wrath is awesome, at times linked metaphorically to words like famine, flood, cursing, conflagration, devouring, reaping, demolishing, slaughtering, smelting, refining, siege, and battle. Little wonder King Solomon tells us "the fear of the Lord is the beginning of wisdom." And it's a wonder anyone can get beyond fear to love.

It appears God's wrath can be directed against pretty much anyone. There are so many examples that I'll refer to just a few representative ones with several other references for you to study on your own.

First of all, you'd think the Almighty would go easy on Israel, his "chosen ones." Far from it. Indeed the most strangely direct and conflicted statement of all comes from the prophet Amos: "You only have I known of all the families of the earth; therefore I will punish you for all your iniquities" (3:2). Moses pleads with this angry God to cut his people some slack: "Why should your anger burn against your people, whom you brought out of Egypt with great power and a mighty hand? Why should the Egyptians say, 'It was with evil intent that he brought them out, to kill them in the mountains and to wipe them off the face of the earth'? Turn from your fierce anger; relent and do not bring disaster on your people" (Ex. 32:11, 12; see also Deut. 9:8; Ps. 74:1; Isa. 47:6; Lam. 2:1; Ezek. 5:15; Dan. 9:16).

Whole other nations and their rulers also feel the heat of God's wrath. The king of Assyria, for example, receives a withering word from the Lord: "Therefore, the Lord, the Lord almighty, will send a wasting disease upon his sturdy warriors; under his pomp a fire will be kindled like a blazing flame. The Light of Israel will become a fire, their Holy One a flame; in a single day it will burn and consume his thorns and his briars. The splendor of his forests and fertile fields it will completely destroy, as when a sick man wastes away. And the remaining trees of his forests will be so few that a child could write them down" (Isa. 10:16–19; see also Gen. 19:24, 25; Ps. 110:5; Mal. 1:4).

And, lest we think that Middle Eastern nations are the major focus of God's disgruntlement, listen to Moses who, perhaps in a dark moment, wrote, "All our days pass away under your wrath; we finish our years with a moan" (Ps. 90:9). Even the world of nature is not spared: "For a fire has been kindled by my wrath, one that burns to the realm of death below. It will devour the earth and its harvest and set afire the foundations of the mountains" (Deut. 32:22). Sometimes ecological destruction is "collateral damage" as God lashes out at the disobedient, "See, the day of the Lord is coming—a cruel day, with wrath and fierce anger—to make the land desolate and destroy the sinners within it" (Isa. 13:9). The Almighty makes it very clear that it is his pleasure or displeasure that controls the world of nature: "By a mere rebuke I dry up the sea, I turn rivers into a desert; their fish rot for lack of water and die of thirst" (Isa. 50:2b). It's enough to make an environmentalist wince. Who is this angry despot? Is he rational? Or is he mad?

Sometimes he seems irrational at least, or maybe mysterious and dangerous. Who can make any sense of his intent to kill Moses? Or of Zipporah's quick-thinking circumcision of her son that apparently placated God's foul mood? (Ex. 4:24–26). And why would the Lord kill poor old Uzzah, who was merely trying to steady the sacred Ark? (2 Sam. 6:6, 7). Was it because Uzzah had a secret agenda, and used the stumbling oxen as an excuse for touching it? At times like these, God appears to be beyond irrational, mysterious, and dangerous.

Rather, it's like he lives in a parallel universe, radically disconnected, emotionally at least, from what he has made. And he certainly appears to be anything but loving.

And yet, maybe this anger, this wrath, is evidence of his love. Maybe he's ticked because he cares. Maybe he's passionate about our behavior because he sees something in us we don't see: our worth. And maybe our worth is somehow tied to, or reflective of, his worth. Maybe he is truly like a parent, a father, and his wrath is discipline "for our own good."

I remember it so well, and I'm sure, so do you: those moments when your dad or mom meted out punishment with the words, "Now, this is going to hurt me more than it hurts you." You didn't believe it. Now that you're a parent, you may even have tried that line on your own kids. The fact is that as a parent, you're sensitive to any breech, however temporary, in your relationship with your children. And, wonder of wonders, it seems that the Maker of the heavens suffers from the same sensitivity. We, his creatures, have the remarkable power to anger and hurt our heavenly Father. The following are just some of the ways we do it.

How to Upset the Almighty

One sure way is to "murmur." This onomatopoetic word, according to the *Oxford Dictionary*, refers to a relentless, but subdued, "expression of discontent." It implies community disgruntlement, for you can't murmur alone. Your *sotto voce* complaint must echo, and be echoed by, someone else's grumbling. And, like the waves of the sea, or the babbling of a brook, the sound goes on and on.

An excellent example of communal dissatisfaction and discontent with God (and his swift response) occurs in Numbers 11. "Now the people complained about their hardships in the hearing of the Lord, and when he heard them his anger was aroused. Then fire from the Lord burned among them and consumed some of the outskirts of the camp. When the people cried out to Moses, he prayed to the Lord and the fire died down. So that place was called Tabeerah, because fire from the Lord had burned among them" (vv. 1–3).

The people, you can be sure, had been complaining about the deprivations of desert wandering for some time. Like water torture their murmurings had become intolerable to their deliverer. So, in anger, he sent a fire to burn, not them, but against them. It spontaneously erupted around the fringes of their encampment. And it was shocking and violent enough that their "complaints about the hardships" readily gave way to "crying out to Moses" for help. The scorched suburb was forever after called "Tabeerah," which in the Hebrew means "burning" or "place of burning." But the camp itself was later named "Kibroth-Haltaavah," which means "graves of lust" or "graves of craving." Why? Because their complaints had offended their Provider; they had "craved other food" (v. 34) and so he sent "a severe plague" (v. 33) that killed many of them. Ingratitude has its price.

Another thing the Lord views dimly is disobedience. There are countless examples in scripture of God's hurt and anger at Israel's failures to obey, but one of the most colorful and succinct is the story of Achan.

The Lord had just given Jericho into the hands of the Israelites (Josh. 6). Jericho, the oldest city in the world, was seen as the "first fruits" of Israel's conquering Canaan. As a symbol of this winning of the portal to Canaan, the Israelites were to give the first fruits of the plunder to the Lord, that is, "all the silver and gold and the articles of bronze and iron" (v. 19). Everything else, including men, women, children, and livestock (with the exception of the prostitute Rahab and all her extended family) were to be destroyed. Any Israelite soldier who kept anything ("the devoted things," v. 18) for himself would be severely judged.

So here comes Achan. In the confusing melee of battle he discovers an elaborate robe, and some gold and silver. He looks about, sees no one is looking, conceals the treasures beneath his cloak, and rushes back to his tent, where he hides the plunder. He then rejoins the battle, no one the wiser.

God, of course, was the wiser, and as far as he was concerned, Achan's disobedience was Israel's disobedience: "the Israelites acted unfaithfully in regard to the devoted things; Achan ... took some of them. So the Lord's anger burned against Israel" (Josh. 7:1). He expresses his displeasure by abandoning Israel's military as they do a little "cleanup" work after the heady victory over Jericho. They send a minor force to nearby Ai and are summarily routed. Joshua, in a bit of a pout, puts the blame on God.

God, for his part, tells Joshua to get out of his funk, up off his face, and address the real issue: "Israel has sinned..." (v. 11). Then through a process of elimination Achan is exposed, resulting in the total destruction of his household. Only after the bodies and property have been burned does the Lord turn "from his fierce anger" (v. 26).

So much more could be said about the Almighty's umbrage with our fickle and faithless behavior. Whether it's our scorn for his word, apostasy, or idolatry, you can be sure that heavenly outrage always follows. *One thing that really upsets our creator is social injustice.* But I think one general point can be made about the spark that ignites a conflagration of anger from above: God's wrath is ultimately aimed at creatures in rebellion to his will. And, because we're all rebels in one way or another, we all need deliverance from the devastating consequences of divine fury. This deliverance the Bible calls "salvation."

The Lion and the Lamb

Which, in a curious way, brings us to Jesus. Even more curious, is Jesus's own mission statement: "I came to cast fire upon the earth..." (Lk. 12:49). The first four books of the New Testament (the Gospels) are all about Jesus. And interestingly, the New Testament begins and ends with warnings about "the wrath to come." Jesus' cousin, John the Baptist, starts it out with a politically incorrect comment to the religious establishment (the Pharisees and Sadducees): "You brood of vipers! Who warned you to flee from the coming wrath?" (Mt. 3:7). Then, as "King of Kings and Lord of Lords," Jesus "treads the winepress of the fury of the wrath of God Almighty" in the book of Revelation (19:15). Also in Revelation is the striking image of people fleeing to hide "in the caves and among the rocks of the mountains" from the "face of him who is seated on the throne, and from the wrath of the Lamb" (6:15, 16).

And who is this "Lamb"? To mix metaphors, he is "the Lion of the tribe of Judah" (5:5). Handel, in his classic work "The Messiah" keys on this "Lamb" imagery, and rightly so, "Worthy is the Lamb, who was slain, to receive power and wealth and wisdom and strength and honor and glory and praise!" (5:12). The entire passage from verse 5 to verse 14 makes it abundantly clear that Jesus is the Lamb. A lamb who is at the same time a lion—a meek creature with the fearful presence and roar of the King of the Beasts. Cuddle this woolly creature at your peril.

And here is a mystery. The "worthiness" of this lamb/lion is rooted in its willingness to be "slain." The elders in the Revelation, Chapter 5, passage sing about this: "You are worthy to take the scroll and to open its seals, because you were slain, and with your blood you purchased men for God... " (v. 9). What's up with this? Why the blood? Why does the author of the book of Hebrews say "the law requires that nearly everything be cleansed with blood, and without the shedding of blood there is no forgiveness"? (Heb. 9:22). Can anyone in the twenty-first century relate to this "bloody religion"?

The Samaritans can. A few years ago, while my family and I were living in Jerusalem, we traveled to Samaria to witness the Samaritan Passover on Mount Gerazim. Samaria, by the way, is seen by most of the world today as part of the West Bank, with Nablus as its major city. The term "Samaritan" referred in biblical times to the inhabitants of Samaria, whereas today it refers to a small surviving group of 200 to 400 people, most of whom reside in and around Nablus. They see themselves, much to orthodox Jewry's chagrin, as the remnant of the kingdom of Israel. Jewish tradition, on the other hand, has always seen them as half-breeds at best, and mortal enemies at worst. (You can read about them in the books of Ezra, Nehemiah, and 2 Kings.) This is why Jesus' famous parable about the good Samaritan had such shock value. In today's terms, it would have been as if a Palestinian from Gaza were to stop and assist a wounded Israeli soldier.

In Jesus' day, Samaritans were persona non grata in Jerusalem, mainly because they had carried on a centuries-old dispute as to where "the mountain of the Lord" was. To Israel, it was Mount Zion. To the Samaritans, it was Mount Gerazim. Remember Jesus' discussion with the woman at the well in John, Chapter 4? Even this wayward Samaritan woman was well versed in the debate over which mountain was the proper place to worship (v. 20). And the dispute lingers, in a vestigial kind of way, to this day.

So there we were, on the windswept top of Mount Gerazim, with a few hundred spectators surrounding an enclosure wherein about three hundred Samaritans had gathered. The Samaritans were clustered in family groupings, and each family had a lamb. I've never seen such lambs. They were perfect in every way, and most had fresh-cut roses woven into their wool. Each lamb was being lovingly cared for with last-minute grooming by the male leader of each family. As they did so, the people looked expectantly over to a large rock where the Samaritan high priest was about to appear. While we waited, a dark red sun slowly set below us, and the wind blew bitterly cold.

Just as the sun was about to disappear, the high priest appeared. He was a frail wisp of a very old man, walking supported on either side by robust, serious-faced young men. They walked him to the stone and then lifted him onto it. He stood, shaking in the chilling wind, and even as the sun dipped below the horizon, uttered a prayer in a high-pitched, quavering voice.

Everyone's attention was on him, or so we thought. But, when we turned our eyes back to the Samaritan families, we were stunned by what we saw. Every lamb was lying on the ground, dead. While we were watching the High Priest, the family heads had silently, soundlessly, undramatically, slit the throats of their sacrificial lambs—now, only 10 feet from where we stood, one beautiful, rose-adorned lamb was already being dressed for the ritual meal to follow. Its blood slowly darkened the ground.

Then another surprise. Suddenly, in the midst of the assembly, a Samaritan man held up a white-gowned infant with fresh lamb's blood smeared on its forehead. The people clustered around and began to praise God with an almost deafening roar.

They went on and on. Indeed, this praise continued for fifty minutes without pause. It was a solid, relentless sound of joy that reverberated from Gerazim to nearby Mount Ebal, and filled the darkening sky. Its depth and richness made us feel like we had been taken back to the days of the Old Testament. It truly was one of the most unique experiences of our lives.

We drove back to Jerusalem, trying to absorb what we had seen, heard, and felt. Our conversation was full of exclamation, curiosity, wonder, amazement, and question. "I was shocked to turn and see those lambs dead! They were so beautiful! They died so quietly, I didn't hear a bleat! The high priest was so old, so frail, so otherworldly! Man, was it windy! What do you suppose was the meaning of the baby? Have you ever heard such singing? I can't believe what we just saw. It's like we visited another planet." Even now, as I recall that conversation, my wonder at what we witnessed has not abated. At the center of that wonder is the powerful, mystical, visual image of an infant held above the heads of the Samaritan families, his forehead smeared with the blood of a lamb.

John the Baptist understood what all the prophet/leaders of Israel had believed right back to the time when God himself provided a lamb for Abraham to sacrifice on Mount Moriah: God's wrath at sin was canceled only by the shedding of a perfect lamb's blood. This is why John proclaimed on the occasion of baptizing Jesus: "Look, the Lamb of God, who takes away the sin of the world!" (Jn. 1:29). He believed, as did his forefathers, that God's justice demanded a penalty for sin. And that penalty was severe—"the wages of sin is death..." (Rom. 6:23). But God is also loving and compassionate: "He is patient with you, not wanting anyone to perish..." (2 Pet. 3:9).

And so, getting back to Romans 6:23, the sentence ends with, "but the gift of God is eternal life in Christ Jesus our Lord." Jesus satisfies God's wrath at sin. He dies in our place. His blood becomes our blood. He is both the infant in the midst and the lamb.

Unlike a lamb, however, and more like a lion, Jesus understood the stakes of dealing with heaven's fury. He felt the full weight of the Almighty's wrath as he hung on the cross. There, just before he died, he cried out the words of Psalm 22:1: "My God, my God, why have you forsaken me?" And, in drinking this "cup" (see Mk. 10:38), he understood that he was delivering mankind "from the coming wrath" (1 Thess. 1:10).

The apostle Paul understood this too: "For God did not appoint us to suffer wrath but to receive salvation through our Lord Jesus Christ. He died for us so that, whether we are awake or asleep, we may live together with him" (1 Thess. 5:9, 10). And, "since we have now been justified by his blood, how much more shall we be saved from God's wrath, through him!" (Rom. 5:9).

Yes, God's lamb had the understanding of a lion, which makes it all the more remarkable that he died willingly without a fight. But this doesn't mean he couldn't roar. Not only was he very angry on occasion (see Mk. 3:5 and Lk. 19:45), but many of his teachings underscored what the Old Testament had taught about God's anger at sin. For example: (a) Those who aren't prepared to meet the Lord will find heaven's gate shut (Mt. 25:1–13); (b) If you don't have child-like faith you'll never go to heaven (Mk. 10:1316); (c) A barren life will be destroyed (Mt. 7:15–23); (d) Living a life independent of Jesus ends in ruin (Jn. 15:1–6); (e) Mislead a child and you'd be better off drowned (Mk. 9:42); (f) Those who don't fear God should fear hell (Lk. 12:4, 5).

This is pretty scary stuff, but there is a happy ending for those who allow the "blood of the Lamb" to cover their sins and mitigate God's wrath. Let's get back to 1 Thessalonians 5:9; in the Revised Standard Version of the Bible it says, "For God has not destined us for wrath, but to obtain salvation through our Lord Jesus Christ." God has enacted a plan in the life, death, and resurrection of the "Lamb" that will culminate in a sinless universe, where a "new heaven and a new earth" will prevail, and "death shall be no more." This coming world will be a world where "wrath" is irrelevant and nonexistent. Why? Because in Christ "the former things have passed away" and everything is new (see Rev. 21:1–4; Isa. 25:8; 35:10).

One final word about "wrath" (then I get back to the "Titan"). Even though Christ in his sacrificial death has provided the means for everyone to be "saved" from heaven's fury, we are required to enter into this salvation by freely choosing to accept and embrace the provision. We can't neglect it or pretend it's not there. If we do, we risk everything: "how shall we escape if we ignore such a great salvation?" (Heb. 2:3). Rejecting God's redemptive work in Christ means facing unprotected "the day of God's wrath, when his righteous judgment will be revealed" (Rom. 2:5). Our core obligation, if we accept this salvation, is that we "live a life of love, just as Christ loved us and gave himself up for us as a fragrant offering and sacrifice to God" (Eph. 5:1). As for where to begin, we can take our cue from the condemned criminal hanging on the cross beside the crucified Savior: "Jesus, remember me when you come into your kingdom" (Lk. 23:44).

All this, of course, is meaningless if God is not angry. Salvation proceeds from wrath. Why? Because "God is love" (1 Jn. 4:16) and "He is not willing that any should perish" at his hand (2 Pet. 3:9). (Not perishing, as some think, at "Satan's hand"—he is merely a garbage man collecting the detritus of God's wrath.) So, heaven awaits those who "fear" the Lord, and hell awaits all others. This is the hope and the offense of the gospel.

Dirty Money

If ever "righteous judgment" were to be revealed in Africa today, most of it would uncover the seamy side of Western commerce. Beneath much of the West's business dealings with Africa is a cynical, smarmy underbelly of dirty money.

According to reports available in the public domain (one excellent source: www.theafricareport.com; CIDcom—Le Groupe Jeune Afrique), about 2 to 5 percent of the global gross domestic product (GDP) is "dirty money." The annual GDP of our world amounts to about $32 trillion per year, meaning that anywhere from $640 billion to $1.6 trillion is gained and hidden in the dark shadows of unscrupulous multinational dealings.

Usually, when we talk about Africa's economic woes, we blame leaders who are guilty of siphoning off funds and storing them in Swiss bank accounts. There's no doubt this is a part of the problem; indeed, Nigeria's president has stated that corruption costs his and other African states upwards of $148 billion per year, or 25 percent of Africa's GDP. This is distressing and unacceptable, reason for anger, justification for strict measures from donors and businesspeople regarding financial accountability structures.

But there is a greater evil still: it's called mispricing. How does it work? Here's how *The Africa Report* (no. 2, March 2006, Jeune Afrique, publisher) describes it:

> The basic principle is to use mispricing to take the money out [of Africa]: overpricing the goods that a country imports or underpricing the goods that it exports. For decades, in Côte d'Ivoire, President Félix Houphouët-Boigny and his friends in the commodity trading companies deliberately underpriced the country's cocoa exports.
>
> For example, if the market price for cocoa is $1,000 a tonne, the mispricers would sell at an official price of $500 a tonne. It is the $500 a tonne price that is officially recorded and is paid through the central bank. But the cocoa is still sold on the terminal markets in Europe for $1,000; the $500 illicit profit is shared between the politicians and traders involved in the scam, and banked offshore.

Then, there is transfer pricing, which generally is rooted in multinational corporations in the West. Here's what *The Africa Report* says:

> The other key technique is transfer pricing. This can only happen within a multinational corporation with a headquarters organization, usually in Europe or the USA, and several subsidiaries, usually in Africa, Asia, or Latin America.
>
> Vehicle assembly plants in Africa are typical of such operations. The multinational company negotiates a multimillion-dollar investment in, say, Angola. The government is happy to have the jobs the new enterprise will create. The headquarters company then sells the components to make the vehicles, at a markup of over 30%, to the Angolan subsidiary. The result is that the Angolan subsidiary makes no money: the headquarters company is the beneficiary, as it takes out its payments on the overpriced components from Angola, usually through an offshore tax haven.

This, of course, exploits the developing country and enriches the multinational, further widening the gap between the rich and poor countries, to say nothing of adding huge weight to the crushing load of poverty breaking the backs of Africa's peasants. And, evil upon evil, take a look at this, also from the *The Africa Report*: "Common to all these transactions—mispricing, drug smuggling, or corrupt payments—is the use of the West's pinstriped army of lawyers, accountants, and company formation agents, the experts who hide ill-gotten gains in offshore tax havens. *About half of all multinational trade is routed through these inherently secretive tax havens*" (emphasis added).

What we're looking at here is a global system of dirty money, laundered, tax-evasive, and blatantly exploitative of the poor. Whether it's organized crime, drugs, counterfeit goods, illegal arms, illegal sale of conventional weapons, illegal oil sales, corruption, mispricing, or transfer pricing, we have an international cancerous tumor in "legal" offshore tax havens that is corrupting our world and ultimately destroying the weakest link, the orphan and the widow.

We should be angry. Very angry indeed. We need to stand up for justice, with no rest until the cancer is removed.

Well, so much for my parenthetic digression to the "dark side." Let's get back to the "Titan."

Psalm 68 has been described as "a grand march through the desert to Canaan," referring both to the scope of the psalm and the reference to a journey from the "wasteland" (v. 7) to "the sanctuary" in Jerusalem (v. 35). It certainly is not a travelogue, but there is a large view in this poem encompassing the victory of the God of Israel over the world, in the context of a history bookended by Mount Sinai and Mount Zion. Larger yet is the distinct emphasis on God, both who he is and what he does. Indeed, God is named thirteen times in the poem, and seven names for God are utilized. You might even say the psalm is all about God, with very little about Israel. It certainly is about his "name."

"What's in a name?" you ask. For Israel, everything. And, as we'll demonstrate, for orphans and widows God's name is crucial (which, as you may suspect, requires another digression).

Earlier in the book I described a visit to a "tish" at a synagogue in Mea Shearim. In the corridors surrounding the central room, scores of Hasidim mingled, many of them Americans, discussing points of doctrine in English. Circulating among several of these discussions, I noted that whenever God was mentioned, they called him Ha Shem.

And, having lived in Jerusalem for seven years, with several rabbis as friends, I knew the reason why.

The Name

Ha Shem means "The Name," which, of course, refers to "God." Orthodox Jews will not pronounce the biblical name of God because to do so means invoking his presence, his very person, which invites death. In the synagogues, when reading the scriptures, they will say *Adonai* ("Lord") whenever they read *Yahweh* (the biblical name of God). Even in casual correspondence, when referring to God, they write "G-d." They have a very high view of "The Name," because for them the question is not "Does God exist?" but "Who is our God?" And the name reveals God himself, which is more than enough reason to be afraid. Yet, even as they "hide their eyes" from Him (see Ex. 3:6), they worship him. Indeed, in approaching worship, you've got to be in awe.

Those who "know the name of God" know that even though he is awful in his power and majesty, he has integrity and can be trusted: "The Lord is a refuge for the oppressed, a stronghold in times of trouble. Those who know your name will trust in you, for you, Lord, have never forsaken those who seek you" (Ps. 9: 9, 10). "'Because he loves me,' says the Lord, 'I will rescue him; I will protect him, for he acknowledges my name. He will call upon me, and I will answer him; I will be with him in trouble, I will deliver him and honor him. With long life will I satisfy him and show him my salvation'" (Ps. 91:14–16). When you're "in the know," you're fearful and hopeful at the same time. God is both terrible and tender, destroyer and creator, final authority and present comforter, warrior and healer, roaring like thunder and speaking with "a gentle whisper" (1 Kings 19:12). His name is mighty among the nations (Jer. 10:6, 7) and "majestic in all the earth" (Ps. 8:1, 2). And, in his quieter moments, he likes to call himself "the Father of Abraham, Isaac, and Jacob." He prioritizes the relational. He "sets the lonely in families" (Ps. 68:6).

In verse 4 of the "Titan" we read, "B'Yah shmo"—"his name is the Lord." The name Yah comes from the Hebrew *havah*, which means "to be" or "become." Yah is a contracted form of *Yahweh*, the name God used when he introduced himself to Moses at the burning bush in the

Sinai Desert. "God said to Moses, 'I am who I am. This is what you are to say to the Israelites: "'I am has sent me to you'" (Ex. 3:14).

Some scholars interpret *Yahweh* as "ehyeh asher ehyeh": "I will be what I will be." Others look to a time before the burning bush, speculating there may have been a primitive god named Ya, and that *Yahweh* is a derivative meaning *Ya-hu* or "O He, O that One!" Whatever the etymological tablet-trail might be, this is the name the Almighty uses both on the occasion of the burning bush and later on Mount Sinai when he says, in the preamble to the Ten Commandments, "Ani Yahweh elohe'cha...": "I am the Lord your God, who brought you out of Egypt, out of the land of slavery" (Deut. 20:2). Which introduces another very important aspect of "knowing the name of God."

The "Name" is rooted in history. Time and again the Lord reminds his people that he is their deliverer: "When Israel was a child, I loved him, and out of Egypt I called my son" (Hos. 11:1); "I am the Lord your God, who brought you out of Egypt..." (Hos. 12:9); "With uplifted hand I said to them, 'I am the Lord your God.'" On that day I swore to them that I would bring them out of Egypt into a land I had searched out for them ... the most beautiful of all lands" (Ezek. 20:5, 6).

This is why the Passover (*Pesach* in Hebrew) is so central to Israel's identity—they are known by the name of their God (Deut. 28:10) and that name is inextricably tied to an historical act of deliverance. And, just so you know, God acts on Israel's behalf in history not for their sake, but "for his name's sake": "It is not for your sake, O house of Israel, that I am going to do these things, but for the sake of my holy name, which you have profaned among the nations where you have gone" (Ezek. 36:22). God has great concern for the holiness of his name. Before he is anything, he is holy. (See all of Ezekiel, Chapters 36 and 37.)

So, the historical tipping point of the exodus thrusts Israel out into the desert, on a forty-year learning curve to learn the name of the Lord. First of all, they know he is a deliverer. Now, in the midst of their four decades of wandering the wilderness, they get to know him as the God of the Covenant. And that God continuously introduces himself this way: "I am the Lord your God, who brought you out of Egypt, out of the land of slavery." In a world of local deities this "covenant God" was new, unique, non-derived, and steeped in history. He was the "Deliverer," the God of the "holy ground," the Majesty of Sinai, the Lover of Israel.

There are, of course, many other names for God in the Jewish scriptures. They deserve a study in themselves, but here they are: *El* is the generic Semitic name for "god" or "deity"—it refers to power, or might, and is sometimes used as a synonym for *Yahweh*; *Elohim* is the plural of *El* but usually used in the singular, "the plural of majesty" as in Queen Elizabeth saying of herself, "We are not amused"; *El Shaddai*, meaning "God, the one of the mountains" or "God Almighty"; *El Elyon*, the "Exalted One" or "Most High" (Melchizedek, who blessed Abram in Gen. 14:18–20 was a priest of *El Elyon*); *El Olam*, meaning "God, the Everlasting One" or "God of Eternity" (originally used at the ancient sanctuary in Beersheba—see Gen. 21:33—but was later attached to *Yahweh*, "the living God" or the "everlasting God"—see Isa. 40:28: "From everlasting to everlasting thou art God"—Ps. 90:1, 2 KJV); *El Bethel*, the "God of Bethel"; *El Roi*, the "God who sees me"; *El Berith*, the "God of the covenant"; *El Elohe-Yisrael*, "*El* the God of Israel"; and anyone's name that has "*El*" in it refers to God (for example, Elijah, meaning "My El is Yahweh"). Then, there are other names used, such as Rock, Father, Brother, Kinsman, King, Judge, and Shepherd. So, not only is there a lot in a name, but there are a lot of names. And seven of them are used in the "grand march."

The Grand March

Now, knowing what we do about both the names and wrath of God, and, for the sake of orphans and widows, let's take a small march through Psalm 68, in bite-sized increments.

> Verse 1:
> *May God arise, may his enemies*
> *be scattered;*
> *may his foes flee before him.*

Verse 2:
As smoke is blown away by the
wind,
may you blow them away;
as wax melts before the fire,
may the wicked perish before
God.

Everything the Lord does and the impact his works have on Israel and the world pivots on "May God arise." As he stands up, the ungodly scurry away like a nest of mice that has been suddenly exposed. They flee in fear. This sovereign act blows human hubris and ambition away as if they were smoke in the wind. The wicked decompose in the face of this angry God, just like wax instantly melts when held close to an open fire. His arising means action—righteous action—and the unrighteous, the unjust, are about to feel the thunder of his voice.

Verse 3:
But may the righteous be glad
and rejoice before God;
may they be happy and joyful.

Verse 4:
Sing to God, sing praise to his
name,
extol him who rides on the
clouds—
his name is the Lord—
and rejoice before him.

The elemental foment of wind, fire, thunder, and rain precipitated by God standing up doesn't faze the righteous. Like the wicked, they too are before God, but instead of being decimated, they are full of joy. The Thunderous One, "who rides on the clouds," is to be praised because "his name [*b'Yah Shmo*] is the Lord." When you know his name, you "rejoice before him."

Verse 5:
A father to the fatherless, a
*   defender of widows,*
*   is God in his holy dwelling.*

Verse 6:
God sets the lonely in
*   families,*
he leads forth the prisoners
*   with singing;*
but the rebellious live in a
*   sun-scorched land.*

So we know his name. But, who is he? What does "I will be who I will be" mean? Beyond etymology, that is. The proximity of "father" and "defender" may suggest that his protection of orphans and defense of widows is close to the core of who he is. In the Hebrew language we see "*Yah ... Av ... Din*"—"I am who I am...Father...Judge." He is the sovereign "I am," the parent "Father," the contending, pleading "Judge." "Father," of course, implies loving relationship. "Judge" implies advocacy and justice. And the entry-level fathering and judging relationship is with the most vulnerable, the most easily preyed-upon, the weakest link in any culture at any time or place in human history—the orphan and the widow.

Yah also has an eye for the "lonely" and the "prisoner." He focuses on the visceral need of both. All the person captured in unrelenting solitude wants is "a household" (Hebrew). And the prisoner, deprived of all human rights, dreams not only of freedom, but of a total reversal of his fortunes, so the Lord provides a house and a family for the solitary, and prosperous freedom for the prisoner. For those who call on his name he is a family and a song. For the rebel, however, he is a "land of drought" (literal Hebrew).

Verse 7:
When you went out before your
*   people, O God,*
when you marched through
*   the wasteland,*

Verse 8:
the earth shook,
   the heavens poured down
      rain,
before God, the One of Sinai,
   before God, the God of Israel.

Verse 9:
You gave abundant showers,
   O God;
   you refreshed your weary
      inheritance.

Verse 10:
Your people settled in it,
   and from your bounty,
      O God, you provided for
      the poor.

Elohim, the Giant God, marches from the East with earth-shaking strides, and encounters his people wandering from the West, at Sinai. As his feet make the ground tremble, his upper body causes the clouds to explode with rain, restoring the fertility of the land, and in its bounty "providing for the poor." Mount Sinai becomes the pivot point of Israel's history, the signature of the Covenant, the historical catalyst for the Torah ("Law"), where Yahweh truly becomes *Elohim Elohe Yisrael* ("God, the God of Israel"). Here the Ten Commandments become the DNA of God's inheritance.

Verse 11:
The Lord announced the word,
   and great was the company of
      those who proclaimed it:

Verse 12:

"Kings and armies flee in haste;
in the camps men divide the
plunder.

Verse 13:

Even while you sleep among the
campfires,
the wings of my dove are
sheathed with silver,
its feathers with shining
gold.

Verse 14:

When the Almighty scattered
the kings in the land,
it was like snow fallen on
Zalmon.

Adonai has a great weapon: his "word." It becomes a song "proclaimed" by a great female chorus (in Hebrew, "the ones proclaiming
it" has a female nuance). God the Warrior has arrived! The "kings and
armies flee." Israel's victory is sweet—so sweet, they enjoy the cool of the
evening and fall asleep "among the sheepfolds," awakening to another
day, watching the doves wheeling in the air, their "wings ... sheathed
with silver ... [and] shining gold" by the dawn's early light. They revel
in the power of *El Shaddai* (the "Almighty") and the ease with which
he "scattered the kings of the land." Why, they fled like snow driven
by a fierce blizzard in the mountains ("Zalmon")!

Verse 15:

The mountains of Bashan are
majestic mountains
rugged are the mountains of
Bashan.

Verse 16:
Why gaze in envy, O rugged
*   mountains,*
*   at the mountain where God*
*   chooses to reign,*
*   where the Lord himself will*
*   dwell forever?*

Verse 17:
The chariots of God are tens of
*   thousands*
*   and thousands of*
*   thousands;*
*   the Lord has come from Sinai*
*   into his sanctuary.*

Verse 18:
When you ascended on high,
*   you led captives in your train;*
*   you received gifts from men,*
even from the rebellious—
*   that you, O Lord God, might*
*   dwell there.*

Today in Israel no one refers to "the mountains of Bashan." Bashan is merely a designated area on the northeast side of the Sea of Galilee. The "mountains" are known as the Golan Heights. The only "majestic" height is about 20 miles north of Bashan and it's called Mount Hermon. Rising to a great height (a little over 9,000 feet above sea level), it is owned in part by Israel, Lebanon, and Syria. It is covered with snow for most of the year, much to the delight of Israeli skiers and snowboarders. Israel commands the pinnacle, and has a high-tech military observation post stationed there, vigilant in the defense of the nation year round (even in the 40 feet of snow in winter!).

Mount Hermon has always been seen as a sacred mountain. Indeed there has been an ongoing debate that the Mount of Transfiguration was Hermon, and not Mount Tabor, which towers over the Jezreel Valley. Nevertheless, if I were the psalmist, I'd surely be referring to Mount Hermon, not the Golan, if I were using the descriptive word "majestic." Maybe the world of the psalmist saw Hermon as part of the Bashan range. Then again, in Hebrew, the word translated as "majestic" is "*Elohim*"; so, the text could read, "A mountain of Elohim is the mountain of Bashan." Whatever ...

Mount Zion, on the other hand ("the mountain where God chooses to reign ..."), is a mere bump in comparison to either the Golan Heights or Mount Hermon. It's a knobby little hill on the southeast corner of Jerusalem. And, in modern Israel, it has even lost its name. Now, the southwest hill is called Mount Zion, and the original southeast location is called the Temple Mount. Historically it was called Mount Moriah, the mountain where *Yahweh Yireh* ("the Lord will see" or "provide") provided Abraham a lamb for sacrifice in the place of his son Isaac. It's also the hill where the Garden Tomb is located, where most Protestants believe Jesus was buried and resurrected.

So the tiny limestone bump called Mount Zion is nothing in comparison to the mighty basalt Bashan range, and yet Bashan is "envious." Why? Because *Elohim* has chosen to live or reign there forever. Bashan's peaks are like a pride of stalking mountain lions waiting to pounce on a solitary rogue lioness who threatens their territory. Indeed, Bashan might prevail, for Mount Zion looks defenseless.

But wait. The "war-chariots of Elohim" have appeared! The Almighty, who stood up at Sinai has now ascended to the height of Mount Zion where, surrounded by billions ("a thousand thousands"—Hebrew) of angels ("the hosts of heaven" 1 Kings 22:19), the "Lord of Hosts" now takes his place. The unrighteous enemies of justice have been defeated; now they follow the Almighty in his "train." These rebels praise him even though the words stick in their throats, and they bring him "gifts." "*Yah Elohim*," the last two words of verse 18, represent the pinnacle of an "arising" that began with God marching like a giant to defeat the armies of injustice. The orphan, the widow, the lonely, and the prisoner rejoice. Righteousness and Justice now rule from Zion, for "the Lord, He is God!" is king.

What follows next is a hymn of praise, a song beginning with *"Baruch Adonai"*—"Blessed be [or "praise be to"] the Lord."

Verse 19:
Praise be to the Lord, to God our
*   Savior,*
*   who daily bears our burdens.*

Verse 20:
Our God is a God who saves;
*   from the Sovereign Lord*
*   comes escape from*
*   death.*

Even though God has ascended to Zion, he is praised first for "daily" bearing "our burdens." Whether you're a psalmist or a psychiatrist, human nature insists on reducing the focus of the God of Hosts to our day-to-day needs. "Forget the big picture, Lord, look at us" (as if we were the center of the universe). "Bear my burdens, Lord, calm my fears. My big fear is death. So, save me from it."

And guess what? Instead of dismissing our childish demands, he accedes to them. He "saves" us. Why? Maybe it's because our childhood eventually becomes adulthood—we pass from a space/time garden to a heavenly one, where we become "the planting of the Lord" (Isa. 61:3). And, to survive the metamorphosis, our spiritual DNA needs to be transformed. Our selfishness, our dysfunctional relationships with God and neighbor, must give way to righteous and just behavior. And, precisely because God is the God of the Big Picture, he responds to those who call on his name and "saves" them from his coming wrath.

Verse 21:
Surely God will crush
*   the heads of his enemies,*
*   the hairy crowns of those who go*
*   on in their sins.*

Verse 22:
*The Lord says, "I will bring
    them from Bashan;
I will bring them from the
    depths of the sea,*

Verse 23:
*that you may plunge your feet
    in the blood of your foes,
while the tongues of your
    dogs have their share."*

The "Scatterer" now becomes the "Shatterer." As a contemporary reader I find this passage a bit much. It strikes me as *meyod primitivi* ("very primitive"—Hebrew). It has the same tenor as a comment made by an anti-Bush demonstrator interviewed by a television journalist during the first Gulf War: "We will take that satan Bush, spread-eagle him to the ground in the scorching desert, and let the dogs eat from him!" It turns the stomach.

But the Hebrew scriptures are very clear: the God of Abraham, Isaac, and Jacob is benevolent to the repentant and ruthless to the unrepentant. He shatters the "hairy" (meaning, perhaps, adult) heads of all enemies of justice. He hunts them down, whether they scatter to the heights of Bashan or the depths of the Dead Sea. When he finds them he destroys them violently. Let the Hitlers, Maos, and Stalins of the world, and all other bullies, thugs, rapists, and despots, take notice.

Verse 24:
*Your procession has come into,
    view O God,
    the procession of my God and
    king into the sanctuary.*

Verse 25:
In front are the singers, after
*   them the musicians;*
* with them are the maidens*
*   playing tambourines.*

Verse 26:
Praise God in the great
*   congregation;*
* praise the Lord in the*
*   assembly of Israel.*

Verse 27:
There is the little tribe of
*   Benjamin, leading them,*
* there the great throng of*
*   Judah's princes,*
* and there the princes of*
*   Zebulun and of Naphtali*

God, the Marcher, the giant who stomped through the wasteland, is now the regal Proceeder. It's as though the wandering Israelites rushed ahead of him to Jerusalem and are now lining the hilltops, standing on rooftops, craning their necks for the first view of the procession. He is about to enter the sanctuary on Mount Zion. Sinai, Bashan, and all other sacred heights are now eclipsed. "*Yahweh Elohim!*"—the Lord, he is God! "Praise him in the great congregation!" The Lord of Hosts is here! And, as you would expect of "I am," he displays his sovereignty and power by having the least powerful of Israel's tribes, Benjamin, leading him up to Zion.

One might ask, in reading of all this jubilation and celebration, "What's going on here?" Is this picture all in the psalmist's imagination? Is he projecting from the present to some future day? Or, did *Yahweh* actually present himself in some visible form, so that the Israelites could see him and be glad?

This would be a good time to take a Bible and read 2 Samuel 6 and Psalm 132.

First of all, the Hebrew text says the "Titan" is a psalm "of David." Authorship of Bible texts is often a point of debate, but let's take the text at its word. King David, the man who dances wildly, naked (but for a loincloth), exposed before the "slave girls of his servants" (David's wife Michal's disdainful observation), is the author of Psalm 68. Why the uninhibited display? Because he's leading the "Ark of the Covenant" back to Jerusalem (2 Sam. 6). And this "ark," this elaborate box, containing the tablets of the Ten Commandments, among other sacred relics, is the very personification of *Yahweh*, the *El* of Sinai. In David's view, and the view of "the entire house of Israel" (v. 15), the procession to Jerusalem was nothing other than the procession of *Elohim* himself up to the sanctuary on Mount Zion.

Even as Moses had declared, "Whenever the ark set out" during the desert wanderings, "Rise up, O Lord! May your enemies be scattered..." (Num. 10:35), he would also say "whenever it came to rest" that it should "Return, O Lord, to the countless thousands of Israel" (v. 36). Later, David would say, "arise, O Lord, and come to your resting place, you and the ark of your might" (Ps. 132:8). I have no authorities to reference here, but it is my sense that this song of praise in the latter half of Psalm 68 is cut from the same cloth. *Yahweh Elohim* has "come to [his] resting place." He has returned "home" and his chosen ones are delirious with joy.

Verse 28:
Summon your power, O God;
show us your strength,
O God, as you have done
before.

Verse 29:
Because of your temple at
Jerusalem
kings will bring you gifts.

Verse 30:
Rebuke the beast among the
reeds,
the herd of bulls among the
calves of the nations.
Humbled, may it bring bars of
silver.
Scatter the nations who
delight in war.

Verse 31:
Envoys will come from Egypt;
Cush will submit herself to
God.

Here the psalmist calls on the God of "power" and "strength" ("the ark of your might"—Ps. 132:8) to do what he has done before. "Rebuke" the "beast among the reeds" (perhaps a reference to Egypt—a crocodile or hippopotamus lying in wait beside the river), humble the despots ("bulls") abusing the vulnerable gentile nations ("calves"), "scatter" the warmongers. And the expectation is that upon the display of this sovereign power from Mount Zion, Egypt will send peace-making "envoys," and "Cush" (Ethiopia) will "hasten to stretch out her hands to God" (RSV). War will end. World peace will be realized. The Lord will be praised.

Verse 32:
Sing to God, O kingdoms of the
earth,
sing praise to the Lord,

Verse 33:
to him who rides the ancient
skies above,
who thunders with mighty
voice.

Verse 34:

Proclaim the power of God,
whose majesty is over Israel,
whose power is in the skies.

Verse 35:

You are awesome, O God, in
your sanctuary;
the God of Israel gives power
and strength to his
people.

Praise be to God!

Here is *Elohe Yisrael* in all his glory. The nations of the world sing his praise, reluctantly at first, but they are overwhelmed and eventually beguiled, if not intimidated, by the "thunder" of his "mighty voice." His majestic power rolls over Israel like storm clouds in the skies, and his holy presence can be felt palpably in his "sanctuary." His manifest, awesome strength empowers and emboldens his people to the point where, in one accord, and with full heart they cry, "Blessed be God!"

I remember hearing an old preacher refer to this psalm as "the history of religion in miniature." Why? Because it starts with God's initiative, "God arising," and it ends with the response of the people, "Blessed be God!" In the process of history from Mount Sinai to Mount Zion God reveals himself, and the people get to know "the name" of their God. At the core of that self-revelation is a powerful truth: God is "a Father to the fatherless" and "a Defender of widows." The "pure religion" that St. James talks about (Jas. 1:27) stoops to the most fragile. The orphan and the widow are the goal of proactive faith and their care the litmus test of true religion. The only religion with integrity starts with God, stoops with God, and stops with God. And the orphan and the widow are the first to bless his name.

"Suffer the Little Children..."

$\mathcal{U}$ NICEF, in a recent publication, *The State of the World's Children 2006*, refers to children as "excluded and invisible." They live "in the shadows," on the margins, out of sight, as if they were miniature lepers living "outside the camp." They're poor and powerless, falling between the cracks of ineffectual and underfunded social services, vulnerable to HIV/AIDs, human trafficking, and recruitment to militias and terrorist organizations.

They often are forced into premature adult roles as laborers and "wives" of dissolute men, precipitating a kind of sexual slavery, often resulting in pregnant little girls with fistulas, a hole between the vagina and bladder or rectum, or both, creating constant leakage of urine and/ or feces. As orphans they have no protector. They have no medicine, no health services, limited access to education, unclean water, little sanitation, poor nutrition, and very little money. Small wonder HIV/AIDS is rampant among them. Every day about 2,000 of them are newly infected with HIV. Every day about 1,500 of them die of AIDS-related afflictions. Indeed, AIDS is reinventing childhood for millions; rather than a time of joy, growth, and wonderment, childhood has become a shadowland of pain, suffering, and despair.

Now, I know that Africa doesn't have a monopoly on human deprivation. Lots of other places around the world have more than their share of suffering. Even here in the West there are people in distress, but at least we have a name. We know who we are. Countless thousands of African orphans have no formal identification.

I remember the time Kathy and I visited a community of children in Malawi. While she talked with a large group of kids, I went over to a small child of about two years who was crawling in the dirt. Naked and covered with skin lesions, he looked more like some sort of abandoned pet rather than a human. I bent down to pick him up, but as soon as he looked at me, he recoiled in terror and began to wail uncontrollably. A small girl of about six years came running over; I assumed she was his sister.

"What's his name?" I asked, as she picked him up and comforted him.

"Baby," she replied to my interpreter.

"I know he's a baby, but what's the baby's name?" I gently prodded.

"Baby," she said, "we call him Baby."

So here's a little guy with no identity. Quite likely his sister has none either. No birth certificate. No record anywhere of their existence. They're invisible, even to themselves.

The "Titan" says God is a "father to the fatherless." As his representative, the Church must take up this role. We Christians in the West must help the African Church help the children. Priority number one: make children visible. We can do this in a number of ways.

Here's what I'm encouraging the African churches to do:

1. *Treat every child as your own.* Identify each child in your catchment area. If they don't have a name, give them one. Make sure they're registered with your local social services and with your church. Create a birth and death register, keep it updated and under lock and key. Let no one pass through life unnoted and unnoticed.

2. *Provide spiritual nurture for each child.* Don't buy into the West's politically correct thinking that says, "We're not to impose faith on a child. Let him decide when he's ready." While we're waiting for him to choose, the neighborhood gang, the encroaching militias, the international terrorist organizations will move into the gap we've left and will powerfully influence his malleable mind. The scripture says we're to "train up a child in the way he should go so that he'll not depart from it" when he's an adult. Children are naturally spiritual. The Church must be their spiritual home.

3. *Become activists in child advocacy.* Children are powerless. They need a defender. Make sure there's proper documentation with their name on it so that in the event of their parents' death, the extended family will not be able to swoop in and take possession of the home, furniture, clothing, and anything else they can get their hands on, forcing the child out onto the street. Make sure the local chief and the local social services know the child by name. Make it clear to these authorities that you're standing with and behind the child's rights. Be a champion of children.

4. *Provide comprehensive care for the girl children who are raped.* We're talking horror on horror here for a little four- or six-year-old child. She'll need medical attention, lots of love, and consistent care for years. Make sure you don't let her down.

5. *Be sure to provide voluntary counseling and testing for children whom you suspect may have been exposed to HIV.* Do it in concert with the social services. Apportion some of your budget for the purchase of inexpensive test kits. Be sure to utilize trained personnel. Leave no one in the shadows.

6. *Teach the children about sex.* Promote abstinence before and faithfulness in marriage. Model it for them. Give them both a standard and people who maintain the standard. Model sexual purity.

7. *Teach gender equality.* Hold men in your community accountable for their actions with regard to women. Show the kids that your church has a high view of women.

8. *Educate them.* Establish simple but effective schools where no fees or uniforms are required. Stay up to date with world events. Give the kids a world view.

9. *Provide surrogate mothers for them.* Monitor their nutrition. Supply food when needed. Make sure they are well clothed.

10. *Provide medical care.* Budget for medicines and regular visits from a health care provider. Make a place in your church services to pray for the children by name when they are sick.
11. *Make fun a priority.* Purchase some footballs. Organize sporting events. Give the children the gift of play and laughter.
12. *Pray for them every day.* Give them a hope and a future. This must be the last generation to bear the burden of AIDS.

Jesus said, "Suffer little children, and forbid them not, to come unto me: for of such is the Kingdom of Heaven" (Mt. 19:14). If the Church in Africa is going to respond to the AIDS pandemic, it's got to start with the children. Love them, love the world. Be the presence of Christ to them—for God is Love.

The Old Testament Prophets Speak on Righteousness and Justice

*L*ike all the other prophets in the Old Testament, Jeremiah stressed that knowing God is more than religious services, solemn assemblies, and praise and worship, which in the absence of righteousness and justice can be hollow and hateful. The vertical must somehow be translated into the horizontal. Those who "know the Name" also need to know the names of the poor.

Jeremiah had especially strong words for King Shallum (also known as King Josiah's son, Jehoahaz) of Judah, and his son Jehoiakim:

¹³"Woe to him who builds his
    palace by unrighteousness,
  his upper rooms by injustice,
making his countrymen work
    for nothing,
    not paying them for their
    labor.
¹⁴He says, 'I will build myself a
    great palace
  with spacious upper rooms.'
So he makes large windows in
    it,
    panels it with cedar
    and decorates it in red.
¹⁵"Does it make you a king
    to have more and more cedar?
Did not your father have food
    and drink?
    He did what was right and
    just,

so all went well with him.
¹⁶He defended the cause of the
poor and needy,
and so all went well.
Is that not what it means to
know me?"
declares the Lord.
¹⁷"But your eyes and your heart
are set only on dishonest
gain,
on shedding innocent blood
and on oppression and
extortion."   (Jer. 22:13–17)

A king who is a materialist, who "builds his palace with forced labor,"
is an unrighteous man regardless of his exalted status and unwittingly
"builds injustice into its walls" (v. 13 NLT). "A palace doth not a king
make," says Jeremiah, and, if the king does "not obey" the commands
of the Lord, his "palace will become a ruin" (v. 5).

And what are those commands? "Do what is just and right. Rescue
from the hand of his oppressor the one who has been robbed. Do no
wrong or violence to the alien, the fatherless or the widow, and do
not shed innocent blood" (v. 3). Unlike his son, King Josiah "did what
was right and just, so all went well with him" (v. 15b). He "defended
the cause of the poor and needy" (v. 16) and in so doing "knew" the
Lord (v. 16b).

In Hebrew, script is written right to left and consonants only are
used (in biblical Hebrew there are "vowel pointings," but these are
omitted, yet assumed, in modern Hebrew). Every word has a three-
consonant root, or *shoresh*. The root for "righteousness" is "*z-d-k*"
(*zedek*) and the root for "justice" is "*s-f-t*" (*shefet*). The nouns are *zadkah* and *mishpat*. *Zadkah* means both "justice" and "righteousness."
Mishpat means "justice."

Zedek is the "gold standard," both in heaven and on earth. It is a high
moral and ethical standard that has its roots in the very character of
God himself. The psalmist tells us that "the Lord is righteous in all his
ways and loving toward all he has made" (Ps. 145:17). Mankind, on

the other hand, is unrighteous: "There is no one righteous, not even one" (Rom. 3:10). There are a myriad of references to the "righteous" in the Old Testament, but that righteousness is always predicated on "right relationship" with the Almighty.

With God, "the righteous Judge," as the foundation, the righteous person is stable and unshakable. Here's how King David saw it:

> ¹Lord, who may dwell in your
>   sanctuary?
>   Who may live on your holy
>   hill?
> ²He whose walk is blameless
>   and who does what is
>   righteous,
> who speaks the truth from his
>   heart
>   ³and has no slander on his
>   tongue,
> who does his neighbor no wrong
>   and casts no slur on his
>   fellowman,
> ⁴who despises a vile man
>   but honors those who fear
>   the Lord,
> who keeps his oath
>   even when it hurts,
> ⁵who lends his money without
>   usury
>   and does not accept a bribe
>   against the innocent.
> He who does these things
>   will never be shaken. (Psalm 15)

You might call this psalm David's "summary of the Law." It resonates with the core value and hope of his life, that "the Lord is righteous, he loves justice; upright men will see his face" (Ps. 11:7). The psalmist's word "upright" in modern Hebrew is *yashar*, which means "straight" or "straight ahead." When a person puts one's trust in the Lord, his/her life is lived in one direction—heavenward—and there is no deviation. Righteousness and justice are both moral compass and far horizon. Just over that horizon is God's "holy hill."

There are three applications of *zedek* generally in the Old Testament. One entails the nature of God and his relationship with the nation of Israel. Another involves the legal status and rights of rich and poor. The third describes the quality of relationship between persons.

As you read the history of Israel in the Old Testament, you see a "Gomer" (Hosea's adulterous wife—Hos. 1:2,3) constantly lurching from unfaithfulness to distress, from distress to deliverance, from deliverance to grateful obedience, and back to unfaithfulness. The weight of the "covenant" between her and the Lord seems to be fully on the divine shoulders. She seems to be stuck in some sort of protracted adolescent rebellion. The "remnant" of the righteous within Israel are constantly embarrassed, and depressed, by this and in need of reassurance that their God will not forget them. Their national security is in jeopardy.

Imagine the relief of these *zadikim* ("righteous ones") then, when the Lord says, "Listen to me, you who pursue righteousness and who seek the Lord; look to the rock from which you were cut..." (Isa. 51:1). He kindly asserts that he "will surely comfort Zion and will look with compassion on all her ruins..." (v. 3). He will not only make her deserts bloom, but he will so thoroughly identify himself with his "people" that "the nations" will benefit from Israel's "law" and "justice" as the personifications of God himself: "The Law will go out from me; my justice will become a light to the nations. My righteousness draws near speedily, my salvation is on the way, and my arm will bring justice to the nations" (vv. 4, 5). Regardless of Israel's temperamental dealings with God, the Almighty will not waver in his covenantal relationship with her. "My righteousness will never fail," he says, "my righteousness will last forever" (vv. 6, 8). Israel's hope is totally rooted, not in her performance, but in the righteousness of Elohe Yisrael, the God of Israel. That's why, despite her unfaithfulness, she can "clothe [herself] in strength" (v. 9), because she truly is strong—she is strong in the Lord. Indeed, "the name of the Lord is a strong tower; the righteous run to it and are safe" (Pr. 18:10). And, even when Israel is unfaithful and God disciplines her through the oppression of foreign armies, it is he "who has created the destroyer" (Isa. 54:16), which means that although Israel weeps for the moment there will be singing in the morning. The righteous God of Abraham, Isaac, and Jacob will never walk away. He knows Israel is hurting, but he also knows that tomorrow he will bring comfort. His righteousness demands it. He must do what he must do.

As to legal status and rights, *zedek* sees everyone, rich or poor, as equal before the law. In the Old Testament people are not only innocent until proven guilty, they are also righteous in their innocence. The Law, mediated by kings, judges, and priests is always seen as rooted in God's character, making righteousness itself (as a kind of personification of God's attribute) God's "presence" in judicial proceedings. So, when a case is brought before the court, it's as though it is brought before the Almighty.

Which means the balances will not be weighted in favor of the rich: "You are always righteous O Lord, when I bring a case before you" (Jer. 12:1).

A good example of rich and poor being on a level playing field comes from the story of Judah and Tamar (Gen. 38). Read it, and, depending on your moral predilections, you'll either dismiss it as too sexual and unworthy of biblical inclusion, or delightfully sexual and reason for religious prudes to lighten up. Before you judge it one way or the other, there's something you need to know.

It's called "levirate marriage." The term comes from *levir*, which means "a husband's brother." Its biblical roots go back to Deuteronomy 25:5-10: "If brothers are living together and one of them dies without a son, his widow must not marry outside the family. Her husband's brother shall take her and marry her and fulfill the duty of a brother-in-law to her. The first son she bears shall carry on the name of the dead brother so that his name will not be blotted out from Israel. However, if a man does not want to marry his brother's wife, she shall go to the elders at the town gate and say, 'My husband's brother refuses to carry on his brother's name in Israel. He will not fulfill the duty of a brother-in-law to me.' Then the elders of his town shall summon him and talk to him. If he persists in saying, "'I do not want to marry her,' his brother's widow shall go up to him in the presence of the elders, take off one of his sandals, spit in his face and say, 'This is what is done to the man who will not build up his brother's family line.' That man's line shall be known in Israel as The Family of the Unsandaled."

This, to say the least, was a touch intimidating. So most men buckled and gave in to the pressure. In Tamar's case, her brother-in-law Onan obeyed the letter of the Law by going to bed with her, but practised "coitus interruptus" to avoid impregnating her. His name has been associated with masturbation, called "onanism" by some, but this is misleading. His sin was not solitary sex, but rather the refusal to preserve the family name.

Essentially levirate marriage was a key element in Israel's social safety-net. It provided three vital societal components: preservation of the family name, protection of the family estate, and care for the well-being of the widow. Interestingly, although long gone from the culture of Israel, levirate marriage is practised by some African tribes today.

So back to the poor widow, Tamar, and her rich father-in-law, Judah. Factor in lust (on Judah's part), quick thinking (on Tamar's part), some practical (on his part) and clever (on her part) negotiation of transactional sex, and voila! You have twins conceived, and an embarrassed patriarch (after all, he wanted to have her killed for her "prostitution," until he found out who the father was!). Ultimately Tamar was vindicated in terms of the law; her vindication was two sons: Perez and Zerah. Her husband's family name would now continue.

The key statement in the story, not only about the level playing field regarding rich and poor, but also about the fulfillment of righteousness, comes from Judah, "she is more righteous than I..." (Deut. 25:26). As this chastened son of Jacob saw it, Tamar was within her rights to act as she did, he was not. There is no comment on male domination, subjugation of women, and sexual politics here; it's merely a matter of who is "righteous" before the law.

When it comes to the third application of *zedek*, the quality of relationships, the justice-seeking element emerges. Both Isaiah and Amos (Isaiah was rich, and Amos was poor) decried the religion-weighted righteousness of God's people. Isaiah captured the situation well, when, in response to the question, "Why hasn't God noticed all the trouble we've gone to in putting on this elaborate fast day in his honor?" (Isa. 58:3), he declares the prophetic word, "Is not this the kind of fasting I have chosen: to loose the chains of injustice and untie the cords of the yoke, to set the oppressed free and break every yoke? Is it not to share your food with the hungry and to provide the poor wanderer with shelter—when you see the naked, to clothe him, and not to turn away from your own flesh and blood?" (vv. 6, 7). "Do this," says the Lord, and "your righteousness will go before you, and the glory of the Lord will be your rear guard" (v. 8).

This elaborate religious festival was an offense to God for two reasons: (a) "in the day of your fast you seek your own pleasure," and (b) you "oppress all your workers" (v. 3, RSV). The "church service" had become just another pleasure-seeking exercise, and even while they were piously praising the Name, they were ruthlessly oppressing their employees. So, pleasure seeking in the house of God amounted to unrighteousness (a low view of God—God as a means to an end), and the exploitation for profit of their workers amounted to injustice (a low view of neighbor—the poor as a means to an end). "Sorry" says the Lord, "until you spend yourselves on behalf of the hungry and satisfy the needs of the oppressed, I won't show up to 'bless' your solemn assembly" (see v. 10). Or, as Amos put it, this time on the occasion of a feast day, "let justice roll on like a river, righteousness like a never-failing stream" (Am. 5:24). Otherwise you'd better get used to the rant from heaven, "I hate, I despise your religious feasts; I cannot stand your assemblies" (v. 21).

Speaking of lost, how lost was the city of Jerusalem and its people in Isaiah's day? As you read Chapter 1 of Isaiah it's hard to believe that the Lord is talking about his chosen ones. Rather than being a people characterized by righteousness and justice, they lived and acted like "Sodom and Gomorrah" (exactly the point in vv. 9, 10—"You're like them, so be them.") The first ten verses read like the graphic description of a corpse, yet this walking cadaver still clings to its religious rituals. The Lord can't take it anymore.

[11]"The multitude of your
    sacrifices —

what are they to me?" says the
Lord.
"I have more than enough of
burnt offerings,
of rams and the fat of fattened
animals.
I have no pleasure
in the blood of bulls and
lambs and goats.
[12]When you come to appear
before me,
who has asked this of you,
this trampling of my courts?
[13]Stop bringing meaningless
offerings!...
I cannot bear your evil
assemblies...
They have become a burden to
me;
I am weary of bearing them.
[15]When you spread out your
hands in prayer,
I will hide my eyes from you;
even if you offer many prayers,
I will not listen.
Your hands are full of blood;
[16]wash and make yourselves
clean.
Take your evil deeds
out of my sight!
Stop doing wrong,
[17]learn to do right!
Seek justice,
encourage the oppressed.
Defend the cause of the
fatherless,
plead the case of the widow." (Isa. 1:11–17)

What an indictment of well-meaning religious people! Let's put ourselves in their place. Suppose some wild-eyed preacher stands in our pulpit and says, "I hate this service, I hate this music, your prayers embarrass me, this whole exercise is meaningless, go away!" You can be sure most of us would leave—loudly! The pastor, or whatever committee had invited this wild man to preach would receive an immediate flood of angry e-mails. Some of us would withdraw our tithes and offerings (a favorite ploy of high controllers). And some of us (predictably) would leave the church and join another. We're offended.

Indeed, we're so offended we can't see our own offense. We can't hear the call from heaven to pursue righteousness and justice (v. 17a). The orphan and the widow are not only invisible (v. 17b), it hasn't even occurred to us that true religion starts, not with a building and a ritual, but with them. The self-pleasuring of the church service must give way to the heaven-pleasing, road-less-traveled, committed care of the weakest link. Barring that, we're just "beating the air."

What follows next in the text is almost always quoted or preached out of context. It's usually used by church-people trying to convince unchurched-people to consider the "error of their ways." When, in fact, the context clearly shows that this appeal is to the church-people themselves.

> [18]"Come now, let us reason
>   together,"
>   says the Lord.
> "Though your sins are like
>   scarlet,
>   they shall be as white as
>   snow;
> though they are red as crimson,
>   they shall be like wool." (v. 18)

As I stated earlier, a true prophetic word always ends on a positive note, and here it is: "You don't have to be glaringly sinful, you don't have to be indelibly tattooed with transgression, you can be as pure and clean as the finest lamb's wool, you can be as fresh as newly fallen snow." The caveat? "If you are willing and obedient..." (v. 19).

"Willing" and "obedient" about what? *About righteousness, justice, and the care of orphans and widows.* "If you do this," says Isaiah, the city of Jerusalem "will be called the City of Righteousness, the Faithful City" (v. 26). Repentance from the neglect of the orphan and widow will see "Zion ... redeemed with justice, her penitent ones with righteousness" (v. 27). In fact, if Jerusalem returns to righteous and just behavior, the day will come when "the law will go out from Zion, the word of the Lord from Jerusalem" (Isa. 2:3). Jerusalem will bear the standard of "true religion"; she will be "a light to the Gentiles."

Scripture References

Old Testament

Genesis 1:27; 4:20, 21; 11:4, 8; 12:3; 14:18-20; 15:6; 17:19, 23; 18:25; 19:24, 25; 21:33; 22, 2; 23:17-19; 38

Exodus 2:6, 16, 17; 3:6, 14; 4:24-2, 6; 19:4-6, 20; 20:1-17, 12, 19; 21:7, 15, 17; 22:21, 22-24; 23:2, 3; 25:23; 32:10, 11, 12

Leviticus 11:45; 19:32; 27:30-32

Numbers 10:35, 36; 11, 1-3, 33, 34; 18:24; 33:3

Deuteronomy 5:15; 9:8; 10:17, 18, 19; 12:5, 7; 13:6-10; 14:28, 29; 16:18-20; 18:13; 20:2; 23:7, 8; 24:17-22; 25:5-10, 26; 26:12, 13; 28:10; 32:3, 4, 22, 39; 34:10

Joshua 6:18, 19; 7:1, 2, 11, 26

Judges 4; 5; 7:15; 10:1

1 Samuel 11:11

2 Samuel 6:6, 7, 15; 14:5, 21; 21:11-22

1 Kings 17:7-24; 19:12; 22:17, 19

2 Kings 25:5

Job 1:5; 5:18; 6:27; 24:3, 4, 17b; 29:12-17

Psalms 7:6-9; 8:1, 2; 9:9, 10; 10:14; 11:7; 15; 18:8, 14; 22:1; 37:28, 30; 39:12b; 50:4-6; 68; 74:1; 89:10b, 14; 90:1, 2 KJV, 9; 91:14-16; 92:9c; 94:2, 6; 110:5, 6; 132:, 8; 145:17; 146:9

Proverbs 12:5; 14:34; 17:6b; 18:10; 21:15

Isaiah 1:9, 10, 11-17, 16b, 17a, 17b, 18, 19, 21-23, 26, 27; 2:3, 4; 6:5; 10:2b, 16-19; 11:1, 4, 5; 13:9; 18-19; 25:8; 28:16, 17; 30:18b; 34:11b; 35:10; 40:28; 42:1, 3; 47:6; 49:6; 50:2b; 51:1, 3, 4, 5, 6, 8, 9; 54:16; 58:3, 3 RSV, 6, 7, 8; 61:3

Jeremiah 7:5-7; 9:23, 24; 10:6, 7; 12:1; 22:3, 5, 13 NLT, 14-17, 15b, 16, 16b; 23:1

Lamentations 2:1

Ezekiel 5:15; 20:5, 6; 22:7b; 34:5; 36:22; 36; 37

Daniel 9:16

Hosea 1:2, 3; 10:12; 11:1; 12:9; 14:2b, 3

Amos 3:2; 5:4b, 21, 24; 8:1-6, 11

Micah 6:7b, 6:8

Habakkuk 2:4

Zechariah 7:9, 13-14

Malachi 1:4; 3:5

New Testament

Matthew 3:7; 5:48; 7:15-23; 19:14; 22:34-40; 25:1-13

Mark 3:5; 9:42; 10:13-16, 38; 12:28-31

Luke 10:25-28; 12:4, 5, 49; 19:45; 23:44

John 1:29; 4; 15:1-6

Acts 2; 17:28

Romans 2:5; 3:10; 5:3, 4, 9; 6:23; 8:12-17, 12-39, 35, 38-39; 12:15; 16:1

1 Corinthians 12:1-3; 12; 13; 14

Ephesians 5:1; 6:2

1 Thessalonians 1:10; 5:9, 10

2 Timothy 3:5 KJV

Hebrews 2:3; 9:22; 10:32-39; 11

James 1:9, 10, 27; 2:5, 8, 9, 14-17, 19, 20; 5:1-5

2 Peter 3:9, 18

1 John 4:16, 20b

Revelation 5:5, 9, 12, 14; 6:15, 16; 19:15; 21:1-4

About
the Author

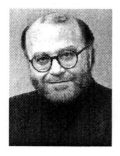

James Cantelon (Toronto, ON) is the founder and President of Visionledd, a Christian charity. Visionledd is working in five southern Africa countries and is about to begin work in Bulgaria as well. James Cantelon is a world leader in the mobilization of churches as a delivery mechanism for pro-active HIV/AIDS work among orphans and widows.

About Visionledd

From www.visionledd.com

"As I stood on the sandy soils of Africa over five years ago, I saw a land with great potential. But the land was trembling on the precipice of the world's greatest disaster.

And I asked, 'Where is the church?'

God birthed in me a dream: that the local churches would become indispensable leaders, activists, and caregivers in the battle against HIV/AIDS. When God showed me the local church, I saw a Mother Teresa. I saw the sick being cared for by the healthy. I saw the North American Church and the African Church working together as partners.

And I understood that God was asking Kathy and me to take the risk of talking with the churches, pleading with them to act.

Visionledd was formed to equip and empower these churches to be the hands and feet of Christ as they minister to the orphans and widows devastated by HIV/AIDS."

OUR MISSION: To motivate, educate, equip and empower compassionate, effective response to the global HIV/AIDS pandemic.

—James Cantelon, founder of Visionledd